ALLE ZEIT WACH
SJ
1842

Oleg M. Eliseev

Cardiovascular Diseases and Pregnancy

Springer-Verlag Berlin Heidelberg New York
London Paris Tokyo

Dr. Oleg M. Eliseev
USSR Cardiology Research Center
3rd Cherepkovskayast. 15a
121552 Moscow, USSR

Translated from the Russian
by Elena Tarkhanova and George Watts

ISBN-13:978-3-642-73607-0 e-ISBN-13:978-3-642-73605-6
DOI: 10.1007/978-3-642-73605-6

Library of Congress Cataloging-in-Publication Data
Eliseev, O. M. (Oleg Maksimovich): Cardiovascular diseases and pregnancy.
Translation of: Serdechno-sosudistye zabolevaniia u beremennykh.
Bibliography: p.
Includes index.
1. Cardiovascular diseases in pregnancy. 2. Heart diseases in pregnancy. I. Title. [DNLM: 1. Cardiovascular Diseases — in pregnancy. 2. Heart Diseases — in pregnancy. 3. Pregnancy Complications, Cardiovascular. WQ 244 E43s]
RG580.C33E4513 1988 618.3 88-8640
ISBN-13:978-3-642-73607-0 (U.S.)

2123/3020-543210

Foreword

Medical science is faced by a number of problems requiring the joint efforts of different specialists. In clinical practice as well, it is often necessary, for the benefit of the patient, to seek advice from a colleague specializing in another field. However, in case of emergency, when one is pressed for time, it is not always possible to consult anyone and the decision to be made becomes the sole responsibility of the physician in charge. In such cases a useful book dealing with the problems of two or more fields of medicine (not always closely related) may prove very helpful. Not long ago pregnancy in women with cardiovascular diseases was considered inadmissible. But women, eager to have children, did get pregnant and gave birth sometimes at the expense of their own lives. At present, the situation has changed. Advances in medical science, technology, and clinical practice have allowed many women suffering from cardiovascular diseases to discover the joys of motherhood. However, it takes an experienced physician, well acquainted with both the cardiological and obstetric aspects of the problem at issue, to determine which of the women are to be the lucky ones.

The author of this book is not only an experienced cardiologist but also an internist well acquainted with obstetric pathology. The book deals with a variety of problems associated with pregnancy in women with heart disease, hypertension, and other cardiovascular disorders, which can occur in pregnant women or women of child-bearing age willing to have children.

To make a decision on pregnancy permissibility in women with heart or vascular disease, the physician specializing in internal medicine (cardiologist or internist) must be well aware of pregnancy-induced physiological hemodynamic changes, changing pathophysiological features of cardiovascular diseases peculiar to pregnancy, and the effect of these diseases on pregnancy. The physician should also bear in mind the possible occurrence of false manifestations of heart disease in a healthy pregnant woman and, in contrast, attenuation or even disappearance of genuine heart disease symptoms and signs during pregnancy. The physician should be able to choose effective diagnostic and, if necessary, treatment methods harmless for the mother and fetus, should know specific ways of managing pregnant women with cardiovascular diseases, and, together with an obstetrician (and sometimes even with a cardiosurgeon and anesthesiologist), should choose an optimal mode of management or together with a gynecologist should also suggest adequate means of contraception to women with a severe cardiovascular disease in whom pregnancy is contraindicated. All this makes the book helpful not only to physicians specializing in internal medicine, but also to obstetricians and gynecologists. Here they will find answers to a number of other questions associated with pregnancy in patients with cardiovascular diseases.

E. I. Chazov, Academician

Preface

During my many years of scientific and practical activity, I have often heard my colleagues (cardiologists and obstetricians) voice the need for a book containing concise information on all the heart and vascular diseases that may be encountered in pregnancy, as well as on obstetric and cardiovascular problems arising in pregnant patients with cardiovascular pathology. After reading books on heart disease in pregnancy or hypertension in pregnancy and respective chapters in handbooks and manuals on cardiology and obstetrics, I could see for myself that the answers to some questions were contained only in one of the books or sometimes only in one of the numerous journal articles. Therefore, I have summarized, my own experience and the experience of numerous of my colleagues from different countries in a book that I hope will be equally useful to cardiologists and obstetricians and that contains not only scientific data but also practical recommendations on the diagnosis and treatment of cardiovascular disorders in gravid females and the management of pregnancy and labor in patients with cardiovascular diseases.

This was not an easy task. I had to combine in one book the information well-known to a cardiologist but not very well-known or practically unknown to an obstetrician and vice versa. In addition, the combination of cardiovascular diseases and pregnancy may give rise to uncommon situations that demand optimal decisions and sometimes prompt action.

It was my intention to help obstetricians adequately assess the role of anatomical and functional cardiovascular disorders for the optimal management of pregnancy, labor, and the postpartal period. But I also tried to make the book useful for cardiologists (internists), to help them clearly understand the threat of pregnancy-induced burdens to women with cardiovascular diseases and what measures must be taken to prevent a fatal outcome for the mother and fetus. That is why some data may seem routine to a cardiologist but not quite familiar or absolutely unfamiliar to an obstetrician, and in some cases, on the contrary, what is evident to an obstetrician will be unknown to a cardiologist. However, in my opinion this will help the two specialists understand each other when they have, in each individual case, to reach a consensus and make a uniform decision on the management of pregnant women with cardiovascular disease; they sometimes must even announce the verdict that pregnancy termination is necessary, or take the responsibility for selecting the optimal method of contraception or sometimes even for sterilization. I hope the book will also prove useful to general practitioners and family physicians whose pregnant patients with cardiovascular diseases certainly seek their advice.

O. M. Eliseev

Contents

1 Introduction

Cardiovascular diseases in pregnant women pose a serious problem both for cardiologists (internists) and for obstetricians. In many developed countries this has led to the institution of specialized clinics or units in hospitals and maternity centers for the management and treatment of pregnant women suffering from cardiovascular and other internal diseases. While in the past termination of pregnancy was recommended in the majority of women with cardiovascular diseases, and women with cardiovascular diseases were in most cases advised to avoid pregnancy and labor, at present the advances in medical science and clinical practice and improved organization of public health services have enabled the majority of women with cardiovascular diseases to experience the joys of motherhood. While physiologists, internists, and obstetricians had recently discussed the problem of nosological forms and degrees of cardiovascular disorders in which pregnancy was permissible under careful medical supervision, today, together with cardiologists and cardiosurgeons, they are discussing problems concerning the management of pregnant women with prosthetic cardiac valves or implanted pacemakers, heart surgery during pregnancy, and the possible impact of various diagnostic procedures and drugs on the fetus.

Nevertheless, cardiovascular diseases represent the most prevalent extragenital pathology observed in pregnant women, and one of the leading causes of maternal mortality, though in the last two or three decades it has considerably decreased.

The data on the incidence of cardiovascular diseases in pregnant women and the cardiovascular mortality rate vary greatly in the statistics of different countries, clinics, and researchers, which to a great extent depends on genuine differences in the incidence of these diseases among women of childbearing age, altered pregnancy permissibility criteria in various cardiovascular disorders, and also differences in the organization of medical care (namely obstetric and cardiological), as well as participation of cardiologists and internists in the examination, management, and treatment of such pregnant women. Moreover, certain authors when determining the incidence of cardiovascular diseases in pregnant women take into account only heart diseases without considering arterial hypertension or vascular diseases.

In recent years the incidence of cardiovascular diseases in pregnant women ranged from 0.32% to 4.7% (Jorde and Morack 1970; Vasilenko 1972; Szekely and Snaith 1974; Persianinov et al. 1978; Nesbitt and Abdul-Karim 1982; McNab and Macafee 1985). In 1927–1968 the cardiovascular mortality rate during pregnancy, at labor, and in the puerperium varied in different countries from 0.4% to 22%, making up 5%–35% of the total mortality in these groups of females (Jaluvka 1970), while in the last 2 decades, despite the diminution in mortality from cardiovascular diseases (Adams 1968; Krayenbühl and Siegenthaler 1974; Serov et al. 1978), this remains the leading cause of death in pregnant women, its relative value still rising with a drop in mortality from other causes, namely, sepsis (Mendelson 1960; Bloshansky 1974). In the United States heart diseases rank fourth as a cause of maternal death (they are exceeded only by deaths from hemorrhages, preeclampsia-eclampsia, and infection). In some large maternity centers cardiovascular disease is the most common cause of maternal mortality (Nesbitt and Abdul-Karim 1982). The highest mortality rate is revealed in pregnant women with cardiovascular disease complicated by pulmonary hypertension. The mortality rate among pregnant women with Eisenmenger's syndrome is 25%–70% (Jones and Howitt 1965; Pitts et al. 1977), it being somewhat lower in patients with severe mitral stenosis also accompanied by pulmonary hypertension. It is noteworthy that patients with cardiovascular diseases in many cases die not during pregnancy, but at labor, in the puerperium, or within the 1st year after childbirth. It should be borne in mind that the onset of hemodynamic shifts during labor and in the early postpartum period is so rapid that little time is left for starting emergency procedures.

The cardiologist (or internist) should consider pregnancy in women with cardiovascular diseases as a severe and long-term load on the affected organ and sometimes as a vital risk factor. Patients with cardiovascular diseases who are under constant care of a physician (a general practitioner or a family doctor, a cardiologist) should be warned about the possible risks associated with pregnancy long in advance, before gestation, and even before marriage. These physicians should assess the permissibility of pregnancy in women of childbearing age and inform the patient of their opinion. When a patient does get pregnant the cardiologist (internist) should once again consider all the "pros" and "cons", and if the decision is positive, the patient should be managed through pregnancy by a cardiologist and an obstetrician, with all the necessary preventive and/or therapeutic measures performed to avert possible complications of both cardiovascular diseases and pregnancy. Women with heart diseases should give birth when they are young, when there are no marked myocardial changes, and when the woman faces less hazards of a congestive heart failure.

Pregnancy is a dynamic process. It is associated with gradual (sometimes sudden) changes in hemodynamics, hormonal status and many other physiological functions. Therefore, it is important to diagnose the case correctly and determine the exact nosological form of cardiovascular disease, its etiology (e.g., myocarditis can be rheumatic, postinfective, allergic, or toxic), and functional state of the cardiovascular system. It is also essential to assess the activity of the primary pathological process (rheumatic fever, rheumatoid arthritis, glomerulonephritis, thyrotoxicosis, etc.) provoking cardiovascular disorders, and to detect focal infection (tonsillitis, sinusitis, cholecystitis, caries, etc.) and concomitant diseases, e.g., anemia and other hematological disorders, and renal diseases.

The management of pregnant women suffering from cardiovascular diseases is often associated with the necessity to solve not only medical but also moral and social problems. Children, as a rule, consolidate the family, while their absence can become the reason for a divorce. In some cases, the desire of a sick woman to have a child and a real family is so strong that she is ready to take an obvious and sometimes unjustified risk. In such cases, the physician not only has to inquire into the patient's history, but also to try to find out her husband's opinion on the problem, often seeking his cooperation in talking the woman into making a rational decision.

In some cases, the woman's desire to become a mother can be realized after successful treatment, which at present is sometimes surgical. In other cases, the physician has to take into consideration the specific situation in the family and take certain risks. Sometimes the physician should firmly insist on adequate contraception or termination of pregnancy.

The above serious, but solvable, problems face a cardiologist (internist) who has to make a decision whether to allow pregnancy and childbirth in a woman with cardiovascular disease without risking her life and health, and the life and health of the fetus and child.

2 Hemodynamic and Cardiac Function Changes in Pregnancy

Pregnancy is associated with physiologically reversible, but rather marked, changes in hemodynamics and cardiac function caused by an increased load on the cardiovascular system and elevated estrogen, progesterone, and prostaglandin E_1 and E_2 blood levels. The load increase is related to intensified metabolism ensuring the vital requirements of the fetus, increased circulating blood mass, the appearance of an accessory placental circulatory system, and finally, a gradual increase in body weight during pregnancy. Enlargement of the uterus leads to limited diaphragm mobility, increased intraabdominal pressure, and changes in the heart position, thus influencing heart function. In pregnant women with cardiovascular diseases, such hemodynamic shifts can prove unfavourable and even dangerous, for they are superimposed on the already existing hemodynamic changes caused by the disease. In some previously healthy women, complications (severe preeclempsia-eclampsia, etc.) may induce serious cardiovascular disorders and pathological hemodynamic changes in addition to physiological shifts. Last but not least, for the sake of the future child, it should be borne in mind that inadequate changes of maternal hemodynamics, having an adverse effect on uteroplacental circulation, can in some cases cause fetal malformations, including congenital heart disease (particularly if there is hereditary predisposition to it).

To differentiate between physiological and pathological hemodynamic shifts and to perform adequate management and treatment of pregnant women with cardiovascular diseases, the reasons, features, and scope of physiological hemodynamic changes should be understood. Without the knowledge of hemodynamic changes occurring in healthy pregnant women it is impossible to assess adequately pathological hemodynamic changes due to cardiovascular diseases.

A long period of gestation is followed by a short, but extremely important, period of labor associated with physical and mental strain and then by a puerperium equally important in view of hemodynamic and other physiological changes. During labor increased expulsive efforts are manifested not only in increased muscle tension but also in a considerable rise in intrathoracic and intraabdominal pressure, affecting heart function and hemodynamics, while immediately after delivery intraabdominal pressure falls and blood is accumulated in the abdominal cavity organs; blood loss during and sometimes after labor also takes place. The physician should know the hemodynamic changes typical of these periods; he should be able to differentiate between physiological and pathological shifts, perform adequate treatment, if necessary, or refrain from intervention, when it is not vitally important (one should always remember that there are drugs that pass through the placental barrier, some of them penetrating the maternal milk).

2.1 Cardiac Output, Stroke Volume, Heart Rate, Left Ventricular Work

The increased cardiac output is considered to be the most significant hemodynamic shift observed in gestation. Its maximum increment accounts for 30%–45% of nonpregnancy levels (Ueland et al. 1969; Sullivan and Ramanathan 1985). Cardiac output increases in early pregnancy: in weeks 4–8 it can exceed the mean cardiac output value of healthy nonpregnant women by 15%. The maximum increase in this variable is observed in weeks 20–24 (according to Metcalfe and Ueland 1974) or in weeks 28–32 of gestation (according to Persianinov and Demidov 1977). The maximum cardiac output increment is associated with a noticeable increase in venous return and intensified right ventricular contractions (Zatikyan 1983). Cardiac output is affected by changes in body posture.

The curves of cardiac output changes in different body postures are not parallel during pregnancy. Maximum cardiac output in the supine position is noted in weeks 20–24 and in the lateral and sitting position in weeks 28–32 of pregnancy. Already in the 20th week of gestation the cardiac output in the supine position is lower than in the lateral position and beginning from weeks 28–32 it is lower than in the sitting position (Ueland et al. 1969). The differences might be mediated by reduced venous return in supine pregnant women due to the inferior vena cava compression by the enlarged uterus. During the last 8 weeks of gestation cardiac output at rest (in all body postures) decreases, being in weeks 38–40 of gestation considerably lower in the supine position than in the 6–8th week after delivery; with the patient in the lateral or sitting position cardiac output is almost normal (Rovinski and Yaffin 1966a; Bader and Bader 1968; Ueland and Hansen 1969) or higher than the normal value (Rubler et al. 1977; Quilligan 1982).

In multiple pregnancy cardiac output increment by week 20 of gestation is higher than in single pregnancy and its antepartum decrease is lower (Rovinski and Yaffin 1966b). In multiple pregnancy cardiac output in the last weeks of gestation exceeds the normal level by 15%, whereas in single pregnancy it exceeds the normal level by no more than 10%, often even reaching the normal value. Maximum cardiac output is 20% higher in multiple than in single pregnancy.

Along with cardiac output increment, an increase in the ejection fraction is observed in pregnancy (Rubler et al. 1977). The cardiac output increment in the first half of pregnancy is mainly caused by an up to 30% increase in the stroke volume. As pregnancy progresses, a certain increase in the heart rate is noted (by 10–15 beats per min in single and by 20–30 beats/min in multiple pregnancy), with the stroke volume decreasing and approaching or reaching the normal levels. Stroke volume, measured in the supine position before labor, appears to be lower than in the 6–8th week after delivery, with the heart rate markedly increased. It should be noted that in some women with single pregnancy no obvious heart rate increase is detected.

During labor pains cardiac output is considerably increased. In healthy women cardiac output can increase by 32% following powerful labor pains or by 19% following weak labor pains (Hendriks and Quilligan 1956), with the increment accounting for 59% during delivery. With the patient in the lateral position, there is a less pronounced rise in the cardiac output during labor pains (Quilligan 1982).

In the early puerperium a decline in the cardiac output is observed (Persianinov and Demidov 1977), thought it can still exceed the normal level by 10%–20% (Burch 1977). The increase in cardiac output during labor is mediated mainly by the increase in stroke volume and to a lesser extent by heart rate increase (particularly during labor pains). On the whole, there is normally a certain increase in the heart rate during labor, while labor pains are characterized by a heart rate increase or two-phase shifts (increase-decrease) and, more often, a heart rate decrease, with the latter shift occurring as a reflex in response to blood pressure elevation. With the woman in the lateral position, cardiac output and stroke volume in pauses between labor pains are greater than in the supine position, the differences between these variables and the heart rate during and in between labor pains being insignificant (Metcalfe and Ueland 1974). This may be related to the fact that venous return in the lateral position is maintained at a constant level, as well as to the fact that the pressure of the contracting uterus on the distal aorta is negligible. Cardiac output in the early puerperium rises by 10%–15%, reaching the normal value a week after delivery.

The rise in cardiac output during pregnancy is not apparently related to increased metabolic maternal and fetal requirements, as it reaches its peak when the fetus is relatively small, and with intensive fetal growth cardiac output diminishes somewhat. Cardiac output increases partly due to contractility-promoting hormonal influences (estrogens and progesterone) and partly due to the appearance of placental circulation functioning as an arteriovenous shunt (resulting in the decline in total peripheral resistance). In this case, despite cardiac output increase, there is a mean BP fall due to a certain decrease in diastolic pressure. Blood volume increase and the afterload reduction caused by the decline in total peripheral resistance may contribute to the increase in cardiac output. During labor pains blood outflow from uterine venous vessels can promote the increase in cardiac output.

The rise in left ventricular work during pregnancy parallels the increase in cardiac output, reaching its maximum increment (33%–50%) in weeks 26–32 of gestation. In multiple pregnancy left ventricular work may be 20%–30% higher than in single pregnancy. The heart work augments with the increase in cardiac output, blood volume, fetal growth, uterus enlargement, and body weight gain.

Near term, left ventricular work reaches normal values in single pregnancy, remaining higher in multiple pregnancy, which puts women with cardiovascular diseases at high risk from heart failure before, during, and after labor.

A dramatic rise in left (and right) ventricular work is observed during labor, especially in the second stage, during uterine contractions (the increment even reaching 100%, or 30%–49% in pause between labor pains). In the early puerperium left ventricular work is almost similar to that observed in the antepartum period. Left ventricular work increment during labor is due to an increase in BP, stroke volume, and cardiac output.

2.2 Blood Volume

The increase in this variable is observed as soon as the first trimester of pregnancy, the value gradually growing (somewhat slower than cardiac output), reaching its peak by weeks 29–36 of gestation or sometimes near term (a slight blood volume lowering, as compared with the maximum value near term is more frequent). Maximum blood volume (BV) increment in single and multiple pregnancy is 30%–50% and 45%–70%, respectively. It is lower in the supine position (like plasma and red blood cell volume) than in the lateral position. This may be attributed to blood accumulation in the pelvic and lower limb veins due to the inferior vena cava compression by the uterus or even to the liquid leakage from the vascular bed into the interstitium, resulting from a sharp rise in hydrostatic pressure in the microcirculatory bed caused by the inferior vena cava compression (Chesley and Duffus 1971). To maintain normal hemodynamics it is essential to recognize that BV increase in gestation is accompanied by the vascular bed volume augmentation at the expense of uterine, placental, and mammary vessels and some extension of the venous circulatory bed.

No significant changes in BV are generally observed during labor; however, the early puerperium is characterized by its marked decrease (by 10%–15%), which is more than could be expected following an inevitable blood loss. The difference between postpartum BV decrease and the amount of blood loss during labor can be 120–450 ml. It is assumed that BV decrease in the early puerperium is caused by blood accumulation in the abdominal cavity organs resulting from an acute fall of intra-abdominal pressure and blood outflow into the injured pelvic and perineal tissues. With a considerable amount of blood accumulated, a postpartum collapse can ensue. In some cases (in women with edema, including so-called internal edema) BV increases immediately after labor or a week later due to a great amount of extravascular fluid entering the circulatory bed which can lead to the development of congestive heart failure or even acute pulmonary edema in women with cardiovascular diseases.

Blood volume increase is mostly due to gradual augmentation of plasma volume by 35%–47%, though red blood cell volume also gradually increases by 11%–30% (sometimes 40%). It results in a peculiar hemodilution with decreased (maximum 33%–38%) hematocrit value and hemoglobin level decreasing from 135–140 g/liter to 110–120 g/liter (Hytten and Leitch 1964), sometimes called physiological anemia of pregnancy (pregnant women often show genuine hypochromic iron deficiency anemia). Circulating hemoglobin volume, markedly decreasing in the first 12 weeks of gestation, then gradually increasing, reaches the normal nonpregnant values at the beginning of the second half of pregnancy and significantly exceeds them near term (Persianinov and Demidov 1977).

Hemodilution, reducing blood viscosity, has a favorable effect on hemodynamics; however, it has an adverse effect on the blood oxygen capacity. Affecting the rate and nature of the blood flow, changes in blood viscosity do have a certain influence on hemodynamics. They can be related mostly to hematocrit value changes. However, plasma viscosity can change with increasing content of macrodisperse (increased viscosity) or microdisperse (decreased viscosity) proteins. As there is a decline in the hematrocrit value during pregnancy, viscosity of the whole blood decreases early in pregnancy. The maximum decrease in blood viscosity is observed in the 22nd–28th week of gestation, while near term blood viscosity approaches the normal level, which can be partially attributed to the increased plasma level of macrodisperse protein fibrinogen. The decrease in blood viscosity as well as hematocrit value reduction are more pronounced in multiple pregnancy (Hamilton 1950; Persianinov and Demidov 1977).

During labor no significant changes have been observed either in plasma or red blood cell volume and hemoglobin value. In the early puerperium the fall in the two former variables corresponds to BV reduction, with a more expressed decrease noted in the latter variable.

The changes in plasma volume are virtually parallel to BV alterations. Red blood cell volume in the first weeks of gestation falls below the normal level and then gradually increases. It is of interest that in multiparas the increase in plasma volume is about 10% higher than in primigravidas and in twin pregnancy plasma volume exceeds the normal level by an average of 67%, i.e., more than in single pregnancy —48% (Rovinski and Yaffin 1965; Persianinov and Demidov 1977). Plasma volume and total body fluid augmentation appears to result from increased plasma renin activity and enhanced aldosterone secretion peculiar to normal pregnancy (Sullivan and Ramanathan 1985) leading to sodium and water retention. These hormonal shifts are probably associated with stimulating estrogen and progesterone effects, with estrogens also enhancing the albumin synthesis.

Central blood volume in pregnancy increases, reaching its maximum by the 25th–28th week of gestation, the increment being 20% in single and 30% in multiple pregnancy. The rise in central blood volume is to some extent related to the augmentation of uterine vasculature and the appearance of placental circulation, but is not parallel to total BV increase, as the major amount of the increased BV is distributed in the venous system.

2.3 Blood Pressure, Total Peripheral Resistance, Venous Pressure

Systemic blood pressure (BP) in healthy pregnant women undergoes insignificant changes. There is a trend toward a certain decrease in diastolic and sometimes (to a lesser extent) systolic pressure, resulting in a slight pulse pressure elevation and mean BP reduction. At the same time total peripheral resistance (TPR) decreases substantially during pregnancy; however, BV increase prevents a considerable BP lowering. Pulmonary vascular resistance in pregnancy decreases. TPR reduction is largely associated with the formation of low-resistant uterine circulation (experimental occlusion of the uterine artery was immediately followed by diastolic and systolic blood pressure elevation), as well as with the vasodilating effect of estrogens and progesterone. TPR reduction and decreased blood viscosity facilitate blood circulation and reduce the cardiac afterload.

Some women in the first and second trimesters of pregnancy reveal a more marked BP lowering, with it returning to the normal level in the third trimester. The most pronounced TPR reduction is observed in weeks 25–32 of gestation.

With the pregnant woman in the supine position, systolic BP does not change significantly, while diastolic pressure, TPR, and pulmonary vascular resistance increase slightly, as compared with values measured in the lateral position. It is noteworthy that blood pressure taken with the pregnant woman in the lateral position is higher on the "lower" than on the "upper" arm, with the difference being quite significant (Comino-Delgado 1984).

In multiple pregnancy BP is a bit higher and TPR a bit lower than in single pregnancy. This could be related to a more marked increase in stroke volume and cardiac output typical of multiple pregnancy.

Labor is associated with a moderate, sometimes even pronounced, rise (especially during labor pains) in systolic and diastolic blood pressure, despite a slight TPR reduction (mostly during labor pains). This seeming discrepancy is explicable, for each uterine contraction is accompanied by total occlusion of distal aorta and/or common iliac arteries which results in the blood, pumped by the left ventricle into the aorta, distributing only in the upper and middle parts of the body. BP in the femoral artery during labor pains is considerably reduced (Bieniarz et al. 1968). In the early puerperium slight BP elevation is observed (Persianinov and Demidov 1977).

In uneventful pregnancy, pressor reaction decreases in response to angiotensin infusion (this may partially explain the absence of BP elevation despite an increase in plasma renin activity) and remains unchanged in response to norepinephrine administration (Chesley et al. 1965). In pregnancy, pressor reaction to angiotensin is probably prevented by a high level of blood plasma prostaglandin E (Bay and Ferris 1979). Marked TPR reduction somewhat decreases the adaptation potentials of the circulatory system and may cause dizziness, syncope, and mild edema in healthy pregnant women and pulmonary edema in women with mitral stenosis resulting from volume overload in the venous part of the microcirculatory bed (and the whole venous system).

Venous pressure measured in the arms of healthy pregnant women does not change significantly (Retzke and Schwarz 1976; Chard and Lilford 1983), while measured in the legs it shows a marked increase beginning from the 5th–6th month, exceeding venous pressure 1.5–2 times in the arms near term. Pressure measured in the femoral vein of a supine pregnant woman is particularly high due to the obstruction of the inferior vena cava by the uterus. In the lateral position venous pressure in the legs decreases, without, however, reaching the normal value (which might be attributable to partial compression of the inferior vena cava). The rise in venous pressure may be one of the causes of the appearance of foot, ankle, and leg edema (mild to moderate) in late pregnancy, as well as subcutaneous vein engorgement in the lower extremities.

The data of finger plethysmography and other methods indicate that pregnancy is characterized by increased distensibility of the venous part of the microcirculatory bed and venules and small veins. The capillary bed extends, with capillary permeability increasing (Chebotarev 1960; McCausland et al. 1961; Hunior 1984).

Venous pressure in the arms increases during the second stage of labor particularly during labor pains, normalizing soon after labor. Central venous pressure also rises during labor; in expulsive efforts it can increase from 2–10 to 60–120 mmHg. Before labor, with the woman in a supine position, central venous pressure is, as a rule, significantly lowered.

2.4 Circulation Time, Pulse Wave Velocity

The arm-to-tongue and the arm-to-ear circulation time changes during pregnancy are insignificant. Circulation time sometimes decreases in the 4th–8th week of gestation and slightly increases by the 32nd week, reaching the normal value or being a bit higher near term. The total circulation time can also be reduced in early pregnancy, but then it gradually increases, reaching the normal value. It continues to grow due to cardiac output and BV increase, before childbirth becoming 14%–16% higher than the basal value. Regional circulation time and total circulation time reflect the linear rate of motion; therefore, blood flow increment, caused by hyperkinetic circulation and almost parallel to BV increase, can be determined only by measuring volumetric flow rate.

Venous blood flow in the legs late in pregnancy is considerably slower with the patient in the supine position. During labor the arm-to-ear and arm-to-tongue circulation time decreases. Regional circulation time and total circulation time are normalized in the early puerperium.

The data on the pulse wave velocity in the aorta are conflicting. In some cases its rise in the second trimester of pregnancy, with a following reduction in the third trimester and another rise near term with a fall in the puerperium, are observed (Schwarz 1964). In other cases, on the contrary, the decrease in pulse wave velocity along the aorta is revealed in early pregnancy and in the second trimester, with the increase by the 29th–32nd week of gestation followed by a reduction near term and another increase in the puerperium (Persianinov and Demidov 1977).

2.5 Intracardiac and Pulmonary Artery Pressure

No marked intracardiac pressure alterations are observed in healthy pregnant women. However, a drop in pressure as well as pressure elevation are sometimes revealed in the right atrium and right ventricle. In the absence of other congestive heart failure symptoms and signs right ventricular end-distolic pressure elevation should not be mistaken for right ventricular failure (Burch 1977). The pressure in the left heart chambers is usually normal in uncomplicated pregnancy. Pulmonary artery pressure is usually reduced due to decreased pulmonary vascular resistance, especially at the end of the first and in the second trimester of pregnancy. A slight rise in the pulmonary artery pressure is sometimes observed.

Right atrial pressure increases during labor pains, the most drastic rise noted during expulsive efforts, partially due to an additional venous blood inflow from the uterine vessels. A parallel rise in right ventricular pressure is observed. Pulmonary artery pressure substantially increases during labor pains and expulsive efforts. Right atrial, right ventricular, and pulmonary artery pressure normalize in the early puerperium.

2.6 Regional Circulation

As pregnancy advances, the most substantial (tenfold and more) increase in the uterine blood flow is observed. Renal (and plasma) flow increases in the first trimester of pregnancy, with the final increment being 25%–35% (25%–50% for plasma flow). By term renal blood flow reaches the normal level. Hepatic and cerebral blood flow show no significant changes, with mammary blood flow increasing. Blood flow to the hands substantially increases from the first weeks of gestation, as well as blood flow to forearms, arms, and legs in the second half of pregnancy (Metcalfe and

Ueland 1974). Enhanced skin blood flow is considered a mechanism of increased heat exchange in conditions of intensified heat production.

2.7 Systolic Time Intervals

No marked changes in the cardiac cycle phases are observed in pregnant women. In early pregnancy the preejection phase is somewhat shortened due to the decrease in isovolumic contraction time, the changes becoming more prominent in the second trimester of pregnancy (Rubler et al. 1973; Burg et al. 1974). The asynchronous contraction time remains unchanged in the first half of gestation and gradually decreases in the second half. In the third trimester of pregnancy the isometric contraction time starts increasing. As a result, the preejection phase either prolongs to normal or, in some pregnant women, exceeds the normal duration before childbirth. The ejection time becomes shorter in the third trimester of pregnancy. In the first half of pregnancy a rise in the intrasystolic index and initial rate of intraventricular pressure elevation is observed. In late pregnancy the two variables become lower, with the myocardial stress index growing (Persianinov and Demidov 1977; Skryabina 1984). The analysis of systolic time intervals in the third trimester of pregnancy with the woman in the supine position reveals a prolonged preejection phase due to the prolongation of the isometric contraction time (which might be attributable to lower venous return in this position), shortened ejection time, and a decrease in the intrasystolic index and initial rate of intraventricular pressure elevation. The changes are typical of a so-called phasic hypodynamic syndrome. With the woman in the lateral position, the isometric contraction time and preejection phase shorten and the initial rate of intraventricular pressure elevation increases, which is believed to be indicative of the phasic hyperdynamic syndrome.

During labor the isometric contraction time and total preejection phase at the peak of labor pains become shorter, with the ejection time being prolonged and the initial rate of intraventricular pressure elevation increased. During labor the myocardial stress index decreases and the intrasystolic index increases. Shifts in the systolic time intervals are retained in the early puerperium, with the duration of systolic time intervals gradually normalizing. However, systolic time interval analysis performed several weeks after delivery may sometimes reveal an increased preejection phase and reduced ejection time. The reasons for these shifts are unknown (Burg et al. 1974).

Pregnancy-induced changes in the systolic time intervals are due to increased (associated with hypervolemia) or decreased preload (due to reduced venous return in the supine position) and may be secondary to TPR lowering. The increased power of myocardial contractions in the volume load during gestation can be related to enhanced myocardial contractility due to direct cellular effects of estrogens and progesterone (Tanz 1963).

2.8 Oxygen Consumption

Oxygen consumption closely related to hemodynamic state, progressively increases in gestation, exceeding the nonpregnant levels by 15%–33% near term (Hytten and

Leitch 1964). This may be due to increased fetal and maternal metabolic needs (increased uterine and placental mass) and intensified maternal heart work. A direct dependence of fetal body weight on the increment in the maternal oxygen consumption has been established. Lower increment in oxygen consumption, as compared with cardiac output increase, may be partially induced by the differences in the peripheral oxygen utilization (e.g., by the uterus and other organs) or, more likely, by redistribution of peripheral blood flow. Increased oxygen consumption during gestation is paralleled by an increase in basal metabolism. Oxygen consumption increases, as compared with nonpregnant levels, by 25%–30% near term (Novy and Edvards 1974; Szekely and Snaith 1974), 65%–100% in the first stage of labor during labor pains, 70%–80% in the second stage of labor, and 125%–155% at the peak of the expulsive efforts (Persianinov and Demidov 1977). In the early puerperium oxygen consumption is still 25% higher than the nonpregnant level. Such a drastic increase in oxygen consumption during labor exposes women with heart diseases to considerable risks. The arteriovenous oxygen difference observed in early pregnancy decreases and reaches the nonpregnant levels at term (Chard and Lilford 1983).

2.9 Hemodynamic and Oxygen Consumption Changes During Exercise and Medical Interventions

Exercise-induced hemodynamic changes in gestation have not been fully investigated and are, according to some available data, similar to those observed in healthy nonpregnant women. The emotional strain of labor and delivery (especially in primigravidas) can cause such hemodynamic changes as heart rate increase and BP elevation. Pain can cause stroke volume and cardiac output increase during labor pains, with anesthesia partly reducing the increase. Mean standard effort causes a substantial increase in oxygen consumption in pregnant (as compared with nonpregnant) women, the differences disappearing in the puerperium. However, according to Kusche et al. (1986), oxygen consumption in bicycle ergometry during pregnancy tends to decrease, as compared with oxygen consumption in the puerperium (especially with greater work loads). An increased amount of oxygen is supplied to peripheral tissues due to a considerable increase in cardiac output on exertion. The exercise-induced arteriovenous oxygen difference is lower in pregnant than in nonpregnant women, which might reflect poorer tissue oxygenation in the absence of a marked increase in cardiac output. There is no oxygen debt in healthy pregnant women after mild exercise (Ueland et al. 1979). It occurs with greater work load, but does not significantly differ from the oxygen debt registered in healthy nonpregnant women after exercise of equal intensity.

It should be noted that in pregnancy oxygen consumption and transport are essential not only during exercise but also at rest. Oxygen transport disturbances have an adverse effect on the size and weight of the fetus and newborn in smoking women, women with anemia, and cyanotic congenital heart disease (McMahon et al. 1966; Novy et al. 1968).

Lactation also increases cardiac load, with the increment being negligible in healthy women, but quite deleterious due to an increased oxygen demand in women with severe heart lesions.

During invasive obstetric interventions, including cesarean section, analgesia and anesthesia have a certain effect on hemodynamics. Under local anesthesia cardiac output increases as labor advances. Spinal and epidural anesthesia (with epinephrine) decreases cardiac output and BP before surgery. Transitory hemodynamic changes in the heart rate, BP, and cardiac output during intubation, extubation, and postoperative awakening can arise with general anesthesia using Pentothal (thiopental), nitrous oxide-oxygen, and succinylcholine. The least expressed hemodynamic changes are observed in epidural anesthesia without epinephrine. Epidural anesthesia with epinephrine generally requires special therapy to correct preoperative arterial hypotension. For this purpose the uterus is displaced, and plasma-substituting solutions are rapidly injected intravenously, this being followed by tight bandaging of the lower extremities and injection of vasopressor drugs into veins in the upper part of the patient's body. All these procedures affect both BP and other hemodynamic parameters (Ueland et al. 1968, 1970, 1972; Metcalfe and Ueland 1974). Hydroxydione sodium succinate (Viadril) is an anesthetic having practically no effect on hemodynamics, which makes it quite useful in labor analgesia and cesarean section in patients with heart disease (Pankratova 1974).

The currently used prostaglandins E_2 and $F_{2\alpha}$ for the induction of labor at term and termination of pregnancy in the 13th–27th weeks do affect the cardiovascular system. But their intraamnional and intravenous injection in appropriate doses causes no changes in the heart rate and BP in either pregnant or nonpregnant women (Karim et al. 1971). Intravenous injection of prostaglandin $F_{2\alpha}$ can first cause a slight attenuation of cardiac contractility — the hypodynamic syndrome (more pronounced in patients with mitral stenosis), which gives way to the hyperdynamic syndrome (Samoylova et al. 1979).

When cesarean section is performed before the beginning of natural labor it is possible to avoid the majority of labor-induced hemodynamic shifts, except for a slight transitory increase in cardiac output. But in late pregnancy venous return can increase dramatically after the extraction of the fetus due to the removal of pressure on the interfior vena cava. This may put females with heart diseases at great risk. Following delivery by cesarean section the elevated venous pressure in the legs falls. Blood loss during cesarean section also causes a decrease in hematocrit values.

2.10 Supine Hypotensive Syndrome of Pregnancy

Supine hypotensive syndrome of pregnancy (syndrome of the inferior vena cava compression), developing in some pregnant women, should not be considered a nosological form. It is rather a manifestation of inadequate cardiovascular system adaptation to the inferior vena cava compression by the enlarged uterus and decreased venous return. Clinical features of the syndrome are BP fall (acute and substantial lowering leading to syncope) in late pregnancy (after the 30th week) with the woman in the supine (and seldom in the sitting) position. The loss of consciousness occurs with BP fall below 80 mmHg. With a less pronounced BP lowering, the syndrome can be manifested in the feeling of air deficit, tachypnea, dizziness, blurred vision, tinnitus, pallor, sweating, and possibly nausea and vomiting.

The syndrome is more frequent in pregnant women with hydramnion, a large fetus, and arterial and venous hypotension (Demidov 1976). In spite of the fact that in late pregnancy the inferior vena cava compression by the uterus (causing venous pressure elevation) is observed in all women, the clinical symptoms of supine hypotensive syndrome are noted only in 10% of pregnant women (Quilligan 1982). In the majority of pregnant women, venous return from the lower part of the body is probably effected partially through nonpaired and spinal veins, while the inferior vena cava compression is not accompanied by hemodynamic disorders. The supine hypotensive syndrome does not usually require drug treatment, it being sufficient to turn the woman to her side. The development of collapse due to inferior vena cava compression is a dangerous complication in surgical delivery, as the cause of this circulatory disorder is not always correctly and timely established, and, therefore, the adequate measures are not performed.

Prominent inferior vena cava compression by the uterus reduces uterine and renal blood flow, causes fetal condition to deteriorate, and decreases the maternal glomerular filtration rate. Premature separation of the placenta can ensue and the conditions are created for the development of thrombophlebitis and varicose vein dilatation in the lower extremities.

2.11 Changes in Heart Size and Cardiodynamics

The introduction of ultrasound techniques has made it possible to assess the effect of pregnancy on individual heart structure motion, and left ventricular and left atrial size and to analyze a number of variables, permitting direct evaluation of myocardial contractility. The majority of variables can also be determined by contrast ventriculography; however, this technique is avoided in gestation. Parallel X-ray and echocardiographic studies of the heart size in nonpregnant women show a sufficiently close correlation between variables determined by these techniques. The data of postmortem examination (Zelenin 1962) and echocardiographic studies (Katz et al. 1978; Hunyor 1984) are indicative of increased heart mass in pregnancy, whereas X-ray findings demonstrate a certain increase in the heart size and volume (Silber and Katz 1975; Quilligan 1982). Left ventricular posterior wall and interventricular septum thickness remain practically unchanged, with absolute myocardial mass (especially in weeks 21–24) and relative myocardial mass (per kilogram of the woman's body weight) increasing. The rate of circumferential fiber shortening and the velocity of systolic posterior left ventricular wall motion progressively increase, starting from the 13th week of pregnancy and lowering somewhat near term (Rubler et al. 1977). The rise in the amplitude of motion of the anterior and posterior walls of the aortic root is also revealed (due probably to stroke volume increase). The velocity of left ventricular contractions during systole remains virtually unchanged, while the velocity of its relaxation during diastole is somewhat reduced in the second half of gestation. The amplitude of mitral valve motion and the velocity of its closing remain practically constant, the velocity of anterior cusp motion reducing in the last trimester of pregnancy (Persianinov and Demidov 1977).

Thus, the increase in the rate of circumferential fiber shortening and the velocity of left ventricular posterior wall motion during systole (along with a rise in the ejection fraction) are indicative of increased myocardial contractility. The enhanced myocardial performance in pregnant women may be the result of inotropic estrogen effect stimulating adenosine triphosphatase influence on actomyosin (Cšapo 1950). However, it is noteworthy that moderate heart rate increase also has an inotropic effect and that a certain reduction in the afterload accelerates myocardial fiber shortening. It could be assumed that increased myocardial contractility enables the heart to cope with higher metabolic load and increased BV.

3 Examination of the Cardiovascular System in Pregnancy

A cardiologist (an internist) often has to take the responsibility of making a decision whether a women suffering from a cardiovascular disease may become pregnant or, if she is already pregnant, whether she may be managed through pregnancy and childbirth without serious risk to the life and health of both the mother and her future child. A similar problem faces physicians during the examination of pregnant women with suspected cardiovascular diseases. The cardiologist and internist also have to consider problems of management and treatment of pregnant women with cardiovascular diseases including those of surgical and obstetric interventions.

In pregnancy, it is often rather difficult to distinguish between false pregnancy-induced signs and symptoms of heart disease and the true signs and symptoms of the disease. Consequently, to avoid possible diagnostic mistakes the primary cardiological examination of pregnant women should be performed in early pregnancy, preferably not later than the 12th week. The examination and management of pregnant women should be based on the principle *noli nocere*, as diagnostic and therapeutic procedures safe for the mother could prove harmful for the fetus. However, this does not imply that pregnant women should not, if necessary, be examined and treated. Damaging iatrogenic effects as well as some acute diseases or exacerbation of some chronic diseases in pregnant women are associated with the greatest risk for the fetus in the first 12 weeks of gestation — the period of fetal organ formation.

In many cases, an accurate and relevant history, documented data of prepregnancy examinations, the current inspection and physical examination data in combination with laboratory findings, and electrocardiographic, phonocardiographic, and echocardiographic data make it possible to reveal cardiovascular disorders in pregnant women. Sometimes, however, physicians are faced with diagnostic difficulties, particularly if the first cardiological examination is performed in the second half of pregnancy. In such cases, diagnosis is sometimes facilitated by such techniques as heart catheterization with Swan-Ganz flow-directed catheter and X-ray examination.

3.1 History

The complaints of pregnant women during examination aimed at detecting cardiovascular disorders are not always helpful for the diagnosis. Up to 45% of pregnant women without cardiovascular diseases complain of increased physical and mental fatigability, weakness, dizziness, "shortness of breath", palpitation, feeling of discomfort, stabbing and pressing pains in the heart area, and inclination to syncope after prolonged standing. These disorders are to a certain extent the result of hemodynamic changes that are not necessarily manifested in these symptoms in all pregnant women. These complaints are most frequent in women with neurotic and psychosomatic disorders (some of them have the same complaints before and after pregnancy), with late menarche, painful menstruations, and artificial termination of pregnancy in history. The age of pregnant women, excessive body weight, and the number of previous parities are insignificant in this respect (Wenderlein 1976). In the second half of pregnancy almost one-third of pregnant women with the above complaints suffer from arterial hypotension, the women with neurotic disorders also dominating in in this group of patients (Rimbach and Heiligenstein 1967). Such complaints could be neglected in the absence of cardiovascular diseases and in normotensive patients (except cases when they are too pronounced and aggravate neurotic disorders in a woman); however, in the presence of hypotension, having an adverse effect on the fetus, treatment should be started.

The patient's complaints of severe headache, dyspnea, cough with blood-streaked sputum, hemoptysis, chest pain, palpitation attacks, and episodes of unconsciousness are of essential importance.

The patient's history may offer useful data on the duration of rheumatic fever, valvular heart disease, the number of previous rheumatic attacks and the time of the last attack, circulation disorders, syncope attacks, the efficacy of antirheumatic, cardiotonic and antiarrhythmic therapy, her parities, the course of previous pregnancies and labors, and ordinary and occupational physical activity tolerance. The data of examinations performed earlier in cardiological or other clinics and hospitals are essential for diagnosis and management of such patients.

3.2 Physical Examination

When examining pregnant women the physician must bear in mind that pregnancy-induced hemodynamic shifts can promote some clinical, electrocardiographic, roentgenological, and other findings simulating the signs of some heart diseases. Sometimes hemodynamic shifts can alter the true signs of the diseases. Both situations seem dangerous, since in the former case hemodynamic shifts can lead to false diagnosis of a nonexistent disease and unnecessary interventions occasionally harmful for the mother and fetus, while in the latter case misdiagnosis of heart diseases can expose the health and life of mother and child to serious risks.

False assumptions can be made during the inspection of a pregnant woman. Mild to moderate edema of the feet and ankles, sometimes of the face and fingers, is quite frequent in the second (less in the first) half of normal pregnancy; it is caused by sodium and water retention, elevated lower body venous (hydrostatic) pressure, and increased vascular permeability with a certain decrease (not always present) of oncotic pressure, and can be mistaken for symptoms of congestive heart failure or renal disease. This, in some cases, leads to groundless therapy with digitalis preparations especially in patients with alleged previous rheumatic carditis in history and cardiac murmurs suggestive of valvular heart disease revealed earlier during physical examination. Sometimes edema could be a symptom of preeclampsia-eclampsia, varicose veins, or thrombophlebitis. In recent years, edema in pregnant women has become less frequent, which in part is due to the availability of diuretics.

In some cases, normal pregnancy can be accompanied by edema and/or other signs and symptoms that can be erroneously attributed to heart failure. Since the venous system in gestation plays a more active part in circulation control due to the increase in BV, normal pregnancy can be accompanied by engorgement of the neck veins, subcutaneous veins of the anterior chest wall, and arms (subcutaneous vein engorgement also occurring on the legs, even in the absence of varicosities), which is sometimes mistaken for symptoms of right ventricular failure (Eliseev 1975). Jugular venous pressure can be elevated during normal pregnancy (Nesbitt and Abdul-Karim 1982).

Slightly accelerated shallow breathing and sometimes moderate dyspnea on exertion or at rest in the supine position, resulting from diaphragm elevation and metabolic shifts, are sometimes mistaken for pathological phenomena and are misleading signs of nonexistent diseases (mitral valve disease, etc.), leading to higher pulmonary venous pressure due to left ventricular failure.

Basal pulmonary rales, misinterpreted as congestive, can be heard in normal pregnancy due to the compression of lung bases by the elevated diaphragm affected by the enlarged uterus and intraperitoneal pressure increase. The rales disappear following a few deep inspirations or coughing (Eliseev 1975). Sometimes the pattern of lung "congestion" is roentgenologically revealed due to enhanced pulmonary blood flow in pregnancy.

Horizontal heart position also caused by diaphragm elevation with lateral displacement of the heart apex is sometimes mistaken for heart enlargement. Due to heart displacement, the apical impulse becomes more diffuse and upwardly and laterally displaced. Systolic pulsation is often palpated in pregnant women along the left sternal border, and sometimes the second heart sound is also palpable in the second intercostal space to the left of the sternum (Metcalfe and Ueland 1974). The heart displacement and increased blood flow cause pulmonary artery distension which roentgenologically looks expanded and engorged. It is sometimes considered a symptom of left ventricular failure. X-ray examination sometimes reveals main pulmonary artery prominence. And, finally, heart displacement also causes a leftward shift of the electrical heart axis in the ECG.

Intensified cardiac sounds and cardiac murmurs first appearing in gestation can be mediated by hyperkinetic circulation. These changes appear in the 12th–20th weeks of gestation and usually vanish in the 1st week after delivery or sometimes before term (Krayenbühl and Siegenthaler 1974). Quite often the first heart sound at the apex is intensified. Splitting of the first heart sound over the heart apex is relatively frequent. Most often the second heart sound is accentuated over the pulmonary area. This may sometimes lead to misdiagnosis of pulmonary hypertension and some heart diseases. Less frequently the second heart sound is accentuated over the aorta. The second heart sound expiratory splitting auscultated in pregnant women is more marked in the lateral position.

Distinct third heart sound is sometimes mistaken for gallop rhythm (this misinterpretation can be avoided by phonocardiographic analysis). A distinct fourth heart sound is considerably less frequent (Cutforth and MacDonald 1966). All these phenomena result from the increase in cardiac output, blood volume, and the force of myocardial contractions (Burch 1977), as well as from changes in heart position.

Systolic ejection murmurs, soft blowing sometimes of moderate intensity, are audible (more often with the patient in the supine position) at the heart apex, over the pulmonary artery area, and along the left sternal border in the third and fourth intercostal spaces. The murmurs can attenuate or vanish altogether in the upright position or upon deep inspiration (Eliseev 1975). These murmurs are sometimes confused with rheumatic mitral regurgitation, obstructive hypertrophic cardiomyopathy, or ventricular or atrial septal defect. The murmurs are associated with intensified atrioventricular blood flow, increased systolic volume and slight dilatation of the heart chambers, pulmonary artery flexion due to heart displacement, blood viscosity reduction, and shortening of the ejection period with systolic ventricular pressure elevation. To avoid possible mistakes, one must acknowledge that organic murmurs are, as a rule, audible both in the supine and standing position on inspiration and expiration, and are intensified with heart rate increase.

Diastolic murmurs can be of different origin. The murmur sometimes heard over the pulmonary area, similar to Graham Stell's murmur, is caused by physiological dilatation of the pulmonary artery in pregnancy. The murmur sometimes audible over the tricuspid valve area is associated with increased atrioventricular blood flow. In some pregnant women early diastolic filling murmur is heard over the apex. The murmurs vanish after delivery, but in pregnancy they are suggestive of pulmonic, tricuspid, or mitral valvular lesions.

Continuous murmurs can also be ausculated in late normal pregnancy. A so-called mammary souffle is detected parasternally over the heart base in the second or third left and/or right intercostal spaces. In the supine position it may become more intensive and accentuated in systole (more often) or in diastole, but vanishes with firm pressure of the stethoscope to the anterior chest wall or sometimes in the upright position. This murmur is caused by an increased blood flow in the mammary arteries. A continuous venous hum can radiate through the supraclavicular fossa to the heart base (a low continuous murmur originates in the jugular vein), is more frequently audible than mammary souffle, and disappears upon jugular vein compression or in the supine position. Despite their extracardiac origin these murmurs are often considered as a symptom of patent ductus arteriosus (Conradsson and Werkö 1974). During the last months of pregnancy and in lactation, a continuous bruit of venous local origin may be heard over the engorged and distended breast. It disappears with pressure of the stethoscope (Metcalfe and Ueland 1978).

At times respiratory arrhythmia is shown in pregnant women without heart diseases, and single premature beats and less frequent short-term attacks of supraventricular tachycardia are noted. In rare cases atrioventricular block can develop.

Syncope accompanied by pallor, excessive perspiration, and bradycardia observed in late pregnancy, with the woman in the supine position (syndrome of inferior vena cava compression), and syncope observed in pregnancy with the woman standing in the upright position for a long time, apparently due to decreased venous return or to vasovagal reaction, can sometimes be suggestive of the Adams-Stokes syndrome.

It is noteworthy that in spite of pronounced pregnancy-induced hemodynamic shifts, it is possible that none of the above symptoms and signs can be discovered in healthy pregnant women; however, at times these symptoms and signs can combine and appear in some healthy pregnant women, whereas sometimes these symptoms and signs are manifestations of a true heart disease. Therefore, cardiologists and internists should thoroughly examine and place the woman under continuous care not only in pregnancy, but in some cases also after childbirth, to correct possible diagnostic mistakes or confirm accurate diagnosis.

Significant symptoms and signs of heart disease in pregnant women are: central cyanosis, markedly engorged neck veins, obvious dyspnea, pronounced heart size enlargement and marked changes in heart configuration on chest X-ray films, harsh systolic and distolic murmurs, pericardial friction rub, persistent congestive pulmonary rales, pronounced disturbances of the heart rhythm, and conduction (persistent premature beats, atrial fibrillation, heart blocks, etc.).

3.3 Electrocardiographic Findings

Electrocardiographic data are essential in pregnancy in the presence of rhythm and conduction disturbances due to organic heart lesions or drug intoxications, as well as in left and right ventricular hypertrophy. No substantial changes are observed on the ECG in normal pregnancy. The most typical signs result from hyperdynamic circulation and heart displacement (Lepp and Karma 1978; Schwartz and Schamroth 1979). They include leftward shift of the electrical heart axis with the corresponding changes in QRS complex, decreased angle between QRS and T axes, ST segment depression, depressed, flattened, diphasic, and inverted T wave in the III standard limb and right chest leads, relatively deep (but decreasing during deep inspiration) Q wave, and flattened, deformed, or negative P wave in the III standard limb lead. It should be noted that pregnant women sometimes reveal right displacement of the QRS complex axis (Carruth et al. 1981), with it far from always being a symptom of heart disease, and sometimes reduced QRS complex amplitude.

The ECG recorded in normal pregnant women as a rule shows sinus rhythm; however, sometimes premature atrial and ventricular beats, short paroxysms of supraventricular tachycardia, and ectopic rhythms are registered. In suspected arryhthmias Holter monitoring is indicated. P-Q and Q-T intervals slightly increase within normal limits in early pregnancy, then gradually decrease. As pregnancy advances, an insignificant narrowing of the P wave and QRS complex is noted. A slight decrease in the time of intraatrial, atrioventricular, and intraventricular conduction is associated with hormonal influences. The duration of ST-T interval in healthy pregnant women remains practically unchanged, with the ST segment located, as a rule, on the isoelectrical line.

During labor especially during uterine contractions and expulsive efforts the P wave and QRS complex are narrowed and the PQ interval is shortened (i.e., the time of intraatrial, atrioventricular, and intraventricular conduction is decreased) and a slight rightward deviation of the electrical heart axis is observed (Persianinov and Demidov 1977). However, during labor and in the early puerperium (as well as during pregnancy), heart rhythm disturbances can be recorded in healthy women; they include atrial (or less often) ventricular premature beats, atrial rhythm, wandering pacemaker, sinus or atrial tachycardia, and incomplete or seldom complete atrioventricular block (Lebedeva and Orlov 1965; Upshaw 1970). Besides these rhythm and conduction disturbances, sinus bradycardia (heart rate 60 and less beats per minute), coronary sinus rhythm, sinoatrial block, and the Wolff-Parkinson-White syndrome are observed during labor in rare cases (Persianinov and Demidov 1977).

3.4 X-ray Examination

Radiation exposure is to be avoided in pregnancy. If X-ray examination is inevitable the woman's abdomen must be adequately shielded with a lead-equivalent apron from X-rays. Chest roentgenography is safer than fluoroscopy; however, short-term fluoroscopy is possible, preferably using an electronic intensifier that considerably lowers radiation. X-ray examination should be excluded in the first 12 weeks of gestation. Repeated X-ray examination should be avoided, if possible. When considering the need for heart or vascular surgery in pregnancy, heart or pulmonary artery catheterization together with blood pressure measurements and angiocardiography are performed. At present it is possible to determine right-heart and pulmonary vascular pressure using flow-directed catheters, without X-ray control. With suspected atriovenous fistulas in the extremities, thrombosis, or embolism of limb vessels, angiography is performed. Abdominal aortography (revealing a potential renovascular genesis of arterial hypertension) is contraindicated during gestation.

As pregnancy progresses and diaphragm elevation takes place X-ray examination of healthy pregnant women usually reveals horizontal heart displacement (upward and leftward) without essential changes in the true heart size (due to changes in the heart position its size may seem increased). Straightening of the left heart border and prominence of the main pulmonary artery is usually considered as a consequence of hyperlordosis of pregnancy (Turner 1975). Heart displacement sometimes causes prominence of the pulmonary conus, and changes in the shadow of the heart and vessels resembling mitral configuration (Jonáš 1960). Due to the engorgement of the pulmonary vessels caused by decreased vascular resistance, their shadow becomes more expressed in gestation.

3.5 Radionuclide Examination

Radionuclide techniques should not be used in pregnancy for hemodynamic assessment, angiocardiography, or differential diagnosis of nephrogenic forms of arterial hypertension and thyrotoxic heart disease. It is noteworthy that some authors (Mazhdrakov and Popov 1976) believe it possible to use isotope renography in pregnant women. The use of ^{131}I-labeled albumin and ^{51}Cr-labeled red blood cells to determine circulating blood volume in pregnant women was reported. However, a long-term follow-up of children born to such women has never been undertaken. But it has been established that radioiodine isotopes are taken up by fetal thyroid after the 12th week of gestation (National Research Council, Committee on the Biological Effect of Ionizing Radiation 1980). As in some cases even small doses of ionizing radiation have a damaging effect on the fetus, BV in pregnant women should be determined, if necessary, by the dye dilution method (Evans blue), which is safe for the mother and fetus (because the dye does not pass through the placental barrier), or by the thermodilution technique. There are also reports on the use of ^{99m}Tc for radionuclide angiocardiography in pregnant women. But ^{99m}Tc pertechnetate crosses the placenta (Jankowski 1986) and may be taken up by the mammary glands during breast-feeding (Berke et al. 1973); ^{67}Ga appears to concentrate in the placenta, but probably with minimal fetal uptake (Newman et al. 1978). However, if unavoidable, contrast angiocardiography is preferable in pregnancy. It should be noted that, according to Dattino et al. (1986), radionuclide scintigraphy of the heart – which is extremely informative in atrial and ventricular septal defects, patent ductus arteriosus, and pericardial effusion and in the diagnosis of hypertrophic cardiomyopathy and early stages of heart failure (by ejection fraction decrease) – poses a lower radiation hazard for the mother and fetus than heart catheterization and angiocardiography.

3.6 Magnetic Resonance Tomography

The absolute safety of the technique and the absence of magnetic resonance mutagenic effect has not yet been proved. A fairly distinct image of a 16- to 20-week-old fetus was obtained in women admitted to hospital for the termination of pregnancy (Smith et al. 1983). This technique does not seem advisable in pregnant women, because the magnetic fields applied (static, rapidly varying, and radiofrequent) are very strong, though it can ensure clear visualization of the heart and vessels.

3.7 Phonocardiography

Phonocardiography in pregnancy reveals virtually the same phenomena as auscultation. The duration of the first and second heart sounds remains unchanged. The interval between the second and third heart sounds increases as pregnancy progresses, with the incidence and amplitude of the third sound decreasing during gestation and again increasing in the early puerperium. During exercise testing the third heart sound is more frequently revealed and its amplitude is increased, during deep inspiration the amplitude of the third sound either reduces or the sound disappears. The dynamics of the fourth heart sound recordings and its amplitude in gestation and the early puerperium are the same as in the third sound. The lower incidence of the third and fourth heart sound recordings near term in the supine position can be attributable to decreased venous return due to the inferior vena cava compression by the uterus. Systolic murmurs are more often recorded in the first half of pregnancy over the heart apex and in the third left intercostal space, while in the second half of pregnancy they are more often detected over the pulmonary area. The murmurs over the heart apex, in the third left intercostal space over the tricuspid valve and the aorta, are usually of low amplitude and duration. The murmurs recorded over the pulmonary area can in some cases be of considerable duration and amplitude.

During labor there is a trend toward shortening of the first and the second heart sound duration, and increase in their amplitude and sometimes their splitting. During labor pains the amplitudes of the third and fourth heart sounds increase and systolic murmurs are recorded more frequently (Persianinov and Demidov 1977).

3.8 Echocardiography

Echocardiography is a noninvasive, fairly objective technique, not troublesome for the pregnant woman and safe for the fetus. Having these advantages echocardiography can be repeatedly used. It is applied for hemodynamic (stroke volume and ejection fraction) and cardiodynamic assessment, determining the dimensions and volume of the heart chambers in systole and diastole, measurement of the aortic root dimensions and ventricular septal and posterior left ventricular wall thickness, myocardial mass determination, evaluation of myocardial function, and visualization of inner cardiac structures (especially when echocontrasting techniques are used). Echocardiography seems useful for diagnosing mitral stenosis (with the determination of the degree of mitral orifice area reduction) and regurgitation, aortic stenosis and regurgitation, cardiomyopathies, mitral valve prolapse, bacterial endocarditis, cardiac tumors, pericardial effusion, and some congenital heart diseases and diseases of the aorta. Echocardiographically determined absolute left ventricular volume during systole and diastole, as well as systolic blood volume, are likely to be a bit higher than the ventriculographic (radiographic and radionuclide) findings. This may be due to the fact that the ellipsoid-shaped left ventricle has two axes (long and short), both measured by angiography. Echocardiography determines only anteroposterior size, with all the calculations based on the value of this size. The Doppler ultrasound technique permits a more accurate determination of cardiac output, in pregnant women as well (Haites et al. 1985). Certain difficulties in the evaluation of cardiac output in the third trimester of pregnancy can be related to heart displacement by a markedly enlarged uterus. However, in this case too M-mode echocardiography allows the determination of cardiac output values, comparable to those determined by the thermodilution technique (Lo Cicero et al. 1985). It is essential that Doppler echocardiography can reveal transvalvular gradients and the degree of regurgitation, and can measure cardiac shunts. For the latter purpose contrast echocardiography can be used (Sullivan and Ramanathan 1985).

3.9 Vectorcardiography

To reveal heart hypertrophy and disturbances of electrophysiological processes in the heart vectorcardiography is sometimes applied (Rybkina 1960). Normal pregnancy causes no vectorcardiographic changes (Tomono et al. 1982).

3.10 Exercise Stress Testing

At present bicycle ergometry and treadmill exercise testing are widely used for the assessment of myocardial functional state. The simplest exercise is Master's two-step test. Bicycle ergometry until a heart rate of 150 beats/min is reached can be safely used in pregnant women. In normal pregnancy, cardiac output, stroke volume, and heart work increase, with TPR decreasing during exercise. Threshold load in pregnant women with congenital heart disease and acquired valvular heart disease is decreased.

3.11 Basal Metabolism. Blood Examination

It is important to bear in mind that normal pregnancy is associated with a moderate increase in the basal metabolism (the body temperature often rises to 37°–37.4 °C), the erythrocyte sedimentation rate is generally increased (often considerably), and moderate leukocytosis (sometimes considerable) with leftward shift of the Schilling index is observed. Blood platelet, fibrinogen, and proconvertin levels increase. Fibrinolytic blood activity is reduced (Quilligan 1982). Both false-positive and false-negative rheumatic tests are detected during gestation.

4 Cardiovascular Diseases and Pregnancy

Cardiovascular disease and pregnancy are not a simple combination of two biological states. Pregnancy and pregnancy-induced changes in hemodynamics, metabolism, water, and electrolyte balance — in gestation total body fluid increases by more than 7 liters (Chard and Lilford 1983), 75% of the amount taken up by extracellular fluid; cumulative sodium and potassium retention reaches 950 and 350 mEq, respectively (Chard and Lilford 1983) — require intensified heart work and often aggravate the course of cardiovascular diseases. Hemodynamic changes and altered immunological status in gestation have a deleterious effect on renal disorders accompanied by arterial hypertension. And vice versa, cardiovascular diseases often complicate the course of pregnancy (preeclampsia-eclampsia, threatened miscarriage, premature labor and other obstetric complications are more frequent) and labor, and have an adverse effect on fetal development (due to hypoxemia or sometimes genetic factors).

Adaptive hemodynamic shifts occurring in pregnancy aggravate hemodynamic disturbances peculiar to most congenital and acquired valvular heart diseases. However, in mild to moderate mitral and aortic regurgitation these shifts are favourable rather than unfavorable and in some forms of acquired valvular heart disease and congenital heart disease some shifts prove favorable and some not (Sullivan and Ramanathan 1985). No disbalance between cardiac load and cardiac reserve is observed as a rule in adequately managed pregnant women with heart disease (except for pregnant women with such forms of the disease in which pregnancy is contraindicated). If such disbalance does occur it entails congestive heart failure that worsens prognosis for both mother and fetus. Therefore it seems essential to estimate cardiac reserve in each pregnant woman. It depends on the patient's age, duration of the heart disease, and functional capacity of the myocardium. It is advisable to establish functional capacities of the heart before pregnancy and then estimate them during regular examinations of the pregnant woman.

Pregnant women with cardiovascular diseases can be divided into two groups. The first group comprises women who in the prepregnancy period have already been suffering from acquired or congenital heart disease (including mitral valve prolapse), hypertrophic cardiomyopathy, essential hypertension, and symptomatic arterial hypertensions of different origin. The second group consists of previously healthy women, who in pregnancy developed preeclampsia, thromboembolism of pulmonary artery or other vessels, dissection of the aorta or coronary artery and peripartal cardiomyopathy. In the first group, pregnancy-induced physiological load is superimposed on the already existing cardiac changes, and may eventually lead to heart failure, when myocardial contractility reserve is wasted. In the second group, heart failure during pregnancy is infrequent.

4.1 Heart Failure

The onset of heart failure during pregnancy worsens the prognosis. The lethal outcome in pregnant women with decompensated (congestive) heart failure is ten times higher than in women with compensated heart failure (Jonáš 1960). The development of decompensation may be caused by recurrence of rheumatic fever, bacterial endocarditis (possibly leading to new heart valve lesions) or infective myocarditis, pulmonary embolism, heart rhythm or conduction disturbances, upper respiratory illness, or systemic infectious diseases. Severe arterial hypertension, preeclampsia, anemia, recurrent thyrotoxicosis, physical and nervous strain, abrupt climatic changes, dietary disturbances, and voluntary changes in daily regimen and treatment protocol can all provoke decompensation.

Clinical manifestations of left and right ventricular (left- and right-sided) failure in pregnancy are common. However, sometimes pregnancy-induced hemodynamic shifts can be mistaken for heart failure (in the presence of cardiovascular diseases as well). It should be noted that in the presence of heart failure a rise in cardiac output is much lower and BV increment much higher than in healthy pregnant women; venous pressure is elevated and circulation time increased. Heart failure in pregnancy is associated with increased extracellular fluid volume, predominantly due to the augmentation of the interstitial fluid volume and to a lesser extent due to plasma volume increase; the analysis of systolic time intervals reveals a cardiac hypodynamia syndrome, extracellular sodium is elevated, while blood plasma calcium is reduced (Borima et al. 1977).

In severe congestive heart failure and impaired cardiac function developing in the first weeks of gestation additional pregnancy-induced cardiac burden can lead to the patient's death. In such cases pregnancy is contraindicated. If the woman does become pregnant, pregnancy should be terminated in the early stages upon intensive medical pretreatment. The problems of preserving pregnancy and optimal management and treatment of pregnant women with cardiovascular diseases should be resolved individually in each case. It should be noted that women with a history of heart failure during previous pregnancy are more inclined to sudden heart failure development during current pregnancy. The most dangerous nosological forms of heart and vascular diseases with respect to heart failure development during pregnancy and labor are severe mitral or aortic stenosis, Eisenmenger's syndrome, and marked coarctation of the aorta (Sokolow and McIlroy 1981).

The likelihood of heart failure development becomes higher after the 20th week of gestation and reaches its peak by the 26th–32nd week, slightly decreasing afterwards. In rare cases the onset of heart failure occurs in the 8th–9th week of gestation. Some authors believe that a different degree of heart failure develops in 50% of pregnant women with valvular and congenital heart disease. At present acute heart failure during labor is quite infrequent. However, the risk of its development becomes higher in the puerperium. In patients suffering from mitral valve disease pulmonary edema is most frequent during maximum hemodynamic shifts, i.e., in the 28th–36th week of gestation and 24–48 h after delivery. Remote risk of death in these patients remains high within the first year after delivery.

The diagnosis of slowly developing heart failure in pregnancy is rather complicated. The manifestations of the developing decompensation may be: tachypnea, marked dyspnea, congestive coughing (sometimes with hemoptysis), moist rales at lung bases persistent on deep inspiration and during coughing, pronounced tachycardia, nocturnal dyspnea, or heart palpitation attacks. A threatening symptom is premature beats of increased frequency in pregnant women with valvular heart disease, as they forerun atrial fibrillation with the following heart failure and thromboembolic complications.

4.1.1 Acute Left Ventricular (Left-Sided) Failure

Acute left ventricular (left-sided) failure before, during, and after labor can develop in the presence of mitral stenosis, aortic insufficiency and stenosis, arterial hypertension (especially during hypertensive crises), severe coarctation of the aorta, and long-standing atrial fibrillation. It can be provoked by physical activity, BP elevation, considerable rise in body temperature due to intercurrent disease, intravenous transfusion of blood or blood substitutes following hemorrhages, sustained refractory tachycardia, and nervous overstrain. Acute left ventricular failure leads to elevated pressure and congestion in the pulmonary veins and capillaries, which in gravid females is manifested in cardiac asthma and pulmonary edema (cardiogenic shock has so far not been recorded in pregnant women during extended myocardial infarction, though cases of myocardial infarction in pregnancy were reported).

Cardiac asthma more often develops at night (however, in acute heart overload it can develop at any time) and is manifested in severe inspiratory dyspnea and wheezing. The patient complains of shortness of breath and experiences a sense of alarm and fear; the attack is often accompanied by coughing with scanty serous sputum. The inspection reveals pallor and sometimes sweating and cyanosis. The patients strive to attain a sitting position and to avoid movements. Respiration is frequent and shallow. Moist and sometimes dry rales at the lung bases are detected (mostly at the back). Tachycardia is usually found, some patients have alternating pulse (alternation of pulse waves of normal and weak filling); blood pressure elevation or lowering can be observed.

Refractory attack of cardiac asthma can turn into pulmonary edema. This is accompanied by a very rapid respiratory rate and exhausting coughing with profuse frothy sputum (often blood streaked). The skin becomes cold and gray-cyanotic, and is covered with cold sweat. Breathing is gurgling. Auscultation reveals bubbling rales over the entire lung field. Marked tachycardia is noted. Some patients with cardiac asthma show a marked bronchospastic component (especially smoking women suffering from chronic bronchitis).

In rare cases there is a combination of cardiac and bronchial asthma. Incorrect differential diagnosis of these two conditions leads to inadequate, sometimes fatal therapy. It should be noted that patients with cardiac asthma always have cardiovascular diseases in their history. The patient has the following symptoms: orthopnea, pallor and acrocyanosis, frequent and shallow breathing, difficulties in inspiration (sometimes also expiration); sputum, if any, is serous and abundant; moist rales are predominantly detected at the lung bases. Patients with bronchial asthma have bronchial and pulmonary diseases in their history; the patient is either in the upright or in the sitting position leaning against the edge of the bed, chair, or table; generalized cyanosis is found, breathing is rare with involvement of accessory muscles, expiration is difficult, viscous and scanty sputum at the end of the attack is noted, and whistling and buzzing rales are detected over the entire lung fields.

4.1.2 Acute Right Ventricular (Right-Sided) Failure

Acute right ventribular failure in pregnant women usually occurs during thromboembolism of the main pulmonary artery or its large branches and seldom during interventricular septum rupture. It results from a dramatic rise in systemic venous congestion and is manifested in increasing cyanosis, neck vein distension, and marked and painful liver enlargement, sometimes accompanied by reflectory vomiting.

4.1.3 Chronic Left Ventricular Failure

Chronic left ventricular failure in pregnant women accompanies the same diseases as acute left-sided failure, and besides occurs in chronic diseases of the myocardium and pericardium. The developing pulmonary congestion is manifested in dyspnea: at first following moderate physical effort and afterwards with ordinary physical activity (dressing, eating) and finally at rest; in tachycardia, coughing, and moist bubbling rales at the lung bases. In severe failure the patients experience relief in the semi-sitting position with their legs lowered. Protodiastolic gallop is the hallmark of ventricular failure. Sometimes an alternating pulse is noted and in some cases presystolic gallop is detected over the heart apex. Chest radiography reveals increased interstitial density of the lungs and dilatation of right and left pulmonary artery shadows.

4.1.4 Chronic Right Ventricular Failure

Chronic right ventricular failure can develop in chronic lung diseases, some congenital forms of heart disease with right ventricular overload, tricuspid regurgitation, diseases of the myocardium, and adhesive constrictive pericarditis. Right ventricular failure can be superimposed upon left ventricular failure, resulting from pulmonary arterial pressure elevation and right ventricular overload induced by severe disorders of pulmonary circulation. Right ventricular failure is manifested in congestion in systemic veins and stable tachycardia. Neck (and often arm) veins are distended and pulsating. Acrocyanosis, lowered skin temperature, and enlargement of and moderate pains in the liver are observed; edema is first more marked by the end of the day and then stable, first appearing only in the feet and ankles and later in the thighs, presacral area, and anterior abdominal wall. In severe right ventricular failure, the fluid is accumulated in serous cavities, causing ascitis, hydrothorax, and (usually mild) hydropericardium. The condition is characterized by oliguria, nicturia, slight albuminuria, and hematuria. Congestive hypertension, congestive gastritis, and mental disorders caused by congestion in the cerebral veins can possibly develop.

4.1.5 Combined Right and Left Ventricular Failure

Combined right and left ventricular failure may be primary in diffuse myocardial lesions or sometimes secondary when right ventricular failure is added to left ventricular failure. Sometimes clinical manifestations of congestion are observed both in pulmonary circulation and in systemic veins, with signs of right ventricular failure predominant.

4.2 Functional State of the Heart

To assess myocardial functional capacity in heart failure the classification of the New York Heart Association is usually used:

Class I. Cardiac disease that does not limit activity. Ordinary physical activity does not cause discomfort. Patient has no symptoms of cardiac insufficiency.

Class II. Cardiac disease that produces slight limitation of activity. The patient is free from symptoms while at rest, but ordinary activity is accompanied by undue fatigue, palpitation, and dyspnea.

Class III. Cardiac disease that produces marked limitation of activity. Less than ordinary activity is accompanied by undue fatigue, palpitation, and dyspnea.

Class IV. Cardiac disease that prevents the patients from carrying out any activity without discomfort. Symptoms of cardiac insufficiency are present at rest, and any activity increases them.

Patients belonging to classes I and II seldom develop decompensation. Though less than 20% of pregnant women with heart diseases are in classes III and IV, the maternal mortality in these patients accounts for 85% or more of maternal mortality from cardiovascular diseases (Nesbitt and Abdul-Karim 1982). These are mainly women of advanced age with long-standing disease and cardiac decompensation in history, as well as patients with severe forms of heart disease, marked heart rhythm disturbances, and recurrent rheumatic and other inflammatory processes in the myocardium.

Pulmonary hypertension accompanying a number of diseases (some forms of acquired heart disease, including mitral stenosis, some forms of congenital heart disease, chronic nonspecific lung diseases) and primary pulmonary hypertension constitute special risks in pregnancy, at term, and in the puerperium. In pulmonary hypertension pulmonary artery systolic pressure can reach 100–200 mm Hg, as compared with 25 mm Hg in normal subjects. Patients complain of dyspnea on mild exertion and cyanosis is detected. For patients with primary pulmonary hypertension, syncope of "unknown" origin and angina-like pains in the chest are characteristic. Auscultation reveals accentuated second heart sound over the pulmonary artery, systolic murmur over the tricuspid valve due to its relative insufficiency, and diastolic murmur over the pulmonary artery due to relative valvular insufficiency. Chest radiography shows right ventricular hypertrophy, prominence of the main pulmonary artery, and distention of the main pulmonary artery and its primary branches with decreased (not always) vascular markings in the peripheral lung fields.

To assess cardiac function in pregnant women with valvular heart disease but without an active rheumatic process, the physicians resort to exercise testing (bicycle ergometry). Maximal heart rate is to be limited to 150 beats/min. In this condition threshold load in mitral disease accounts for 60–80 W. In functional classes II and III exercise tolerance decreases to 40–60 W, and in functional class IV to 10–35 W (Vanina 1979).

The estimation of myocardial functional state and its reserve should be carried out with consideration of cardiac and vascular loads not only during pregnancy, labor, and puerperium, but also during possible obstetric interventions aimed at stimulation of labor or termination of pregnancy. Indications and possibilities for cardiac surgery and surgical tactics in pregnant patients with heart disease pose a special and serious problem.

The above facts necessitate constant cooperation between a cardiologist or internist, cardiosurgeon and obstetrician, and, if necessary, anesthesiologist. Joint discussions and decisions (of a cardiologist and an obstetrician) as to the management of labor in women with cardiovascular diseases are of special importance. Standard approaches in these cases may sometimes prove unsafe.

In pregnant women suffering from cardiovascular diseases all the additional factors demanding increased heart work should be avoided, e.g., excessive physical load, mental overstrain and stress, and acute infections, especially those accompanied by body temperature elevation. Foci of chronic infection (tonsillitis, sinusitis, cholecystitis, periodontitis, pulpitis, etc.) should be eliminated. Anemia leading to a rise in cardiac output and heart rate should be treated (oral administration of iron preparations and folic acid not only elevates hemoglobin blood level but also increases blood oxygen capacity). The patients should be treated for arterial hypertension, irrespective of its origin (essential hypertension, coarctation of the aorta, renal disease, or preeclampsia), as hypertension in pregnancy increases the risk of cardiac failure, hypertensive encephalopathy, and aortic dissection. It was found that at least half of the cases of aortic dissection in women occur in pregnancy, though it is not always associated with arterial hypertension (Sokolow and McIlroy 1981). Such diseases as pneumonia and exudative pleuritis can also be the causes of heart failure.

An abrupt increase in cardiovascular load takes place during labor (especially in the second stage). It is induced by uterine and skeletal muscle contractions during expulsive efforts, emotional strain, pains, increased venous return, stroke volume and cardiac output, and elevated arterial and venous pressure. Cardiac adaptation to abruptly increasing load is impeded by its instability: heart work during labor pains and expulsive efforts markedly increases, and slightly decreases during pauses. In patients with cardiovascular diseases this may lead to breakdown of circulatory compensation and the onset of acute heart failure.

If the increase in the venous return during labor pains is not followed by an adequate rise in cardiac output, right-sided heart dysfunction can produce a more marked congestion in systemic circulation and the onset of collapse, while left-sided heart dysfunction can lead to pulmonary edema.

Blood pressure elevation during labor can be the cause of hypertensive encephalopathy, eclampsia, cerebral hemorrhages in pregnant women with arterial hypertension, dissection or rupture of the aorta or one of the arteries (including coronary artery) in the presence of aneurysm.

The risks associated with abrupt hemodynamic shifts in pregnant women with cardiovascular diseases make it essential to decrease the hemodynamic burden of labor. This can be achieved by psychological training, analgesia, rational management of labor with elective shortening of its second stage. Following the delivery all the women with cardiovascular diseases should be carefully examined by a cardiologist.

4.3 Effects of Maternal Heart Disease on the Fetus

The fetal mortality rate in mothers suffering from heart diseases and especially in women with atrial fibrillation is 3%–9% and 50%, respectively (Hamilton 1947; Mendelson 1960). Women with cyanotic heart disease have a high level of spontaneous abortions due to hypoxia. Pregnant women with other forms of congenital heart disease or chronic rheumatic valvular disease often have signs of threatened abortion or premature labor. In pregnant women with prosthetic cardiac valves anticoagulant therapy is associated with a high risk for the fetus. In the case of heart failure developing in gestation the risk of fetal death is three times higher than in heart disease without heart failure. But the risk for the children is not limited by intrauterine, intrapartum, or postpartum death: the frequency of cardiovascular diseases in children of parents with congenital heart valvular disease is six times higher than in those of healthy parents (Hausen and Loch 1973; Metcalfe and Ueland 1978). Children with congenital heart disease are particularly often born to mothers with ventricular septal defect (Protopopova 1981). As nowadays an increasing number of postoperative cardiac patients do give birth, the number of newborns with heart malformations has increased. Congenital heart lesions are detected in 16.1% of babies born to mothers with congenital heart disease (Whittemore et al. 1982).

4.4 Influence of Age and Intercurrent Diseases on the Course of Pregnancy in Patients with Cardiovascular Disease

Women with cardiovascular diseases are recommended to give birth (in the absence of contraindications) when they are young. Cardiovascular disorders in pregnant patients constitute a greater threat for multigravidas, especially those over 30 years of age, than in primigravidas. Prepregnancy assessment of functional cardiac capacity, timely surgical intervention if this is indicated, careful follow-up, and adequate management of patients through pregnancy, during labor, and in the puerperium can prevent cardiovascular complications associated with the burden caused by pregnancy and labor. However, acute respiratory and other intercurrent diseases, sudden onset of atrial fibrillation, and other severe heart rhythm disturbances can complicate a so far uneventful pregnancy in women with cardiovascular diseases. Therefore, such disorders and complications demand adequate therapy or prevention in case of epidemic situations (influenza, intestinal infections).

4.5 Pregnancy and Rheumatism

Pregnancy as such does not necessarily stimulate the recurrence of acute rheumatic fever, but if acute rheumatic carditis first appears in pregnancy the risk of maternal and fetal death increases (Sullivan and Ramanathan 1985). Acute rheumatic carditis may become the cause of sudden death during labor or in the early puerperium even in the absence of an evident valvular heart disease (Szekeli and Snaith 1974). In the presence of rheumatic heart disease acute carditis may provoke the onset of heart failure or aggravate the existing cardiac decompensation. In recent years a trend has sometimes been observed towards overestimation of the potential effects of drug therapy and surgery in the treatment of rheumatic valvular heart disease during pregnancy. This, in some cases, leads to a situation when the physicians allow pregnancy in patients suffering from rather severe heart disease provided therapy is performed, or the patients themselves take such a decision contrary to the physician's advice. This results in the increase of not only antepartum and intrapartum but also remote postpartum (2 months–6 years) mortality (5%–7.6%), worsening of the patient's condition (47.3%), and postdelivery disability of patients with mixed stenosis and mitral valve regurgitation with predominance of stenosis and patients with combined mitral and aortic valve disease (14.3%) (Davydov et al. 1977). Worsening of the patient's condition is most frequently (66% of cases) observed following delivery in patients who suffered from recurrent rheumatic fever or marked heart failure during pregnancy. Most severe circulation disorders are observed in pregnant women who in the prepregnancy period suffered from episodes of heart failure and repeated rheumatic attacks. Recurrent rheumatic fever can be frequently accompanied by pulmonary edema, pneumonia, thrombophlebitis, pulmonary infarction, premature labor, and preeclampsia.

The diagnosis of the current rheumatic process in the presence of valvular heart disease is associated with certain difficulties in gestation and is a matter of utmost importance. The decision on the possibility to advance pregnancy or the necessity of its termination, and on the need for antirheumatic therapy and the choice of the optimal mode of delivery should be based on the presence or absence of an active rheumatic process. The data on the incidence of active rheumatic fever in pregnant women are even more controversial than the data on the incidence of congenital heart and acquired valvular heart disease. Zakirov et al. (1979) have detected an active rheumatic process in 63.8% of pregnant women suffering from rheumatic heart disease, while Vasilenko (1972) only in 1% of such patients. Other authors report that recurrence of rheumatic fever occurs in 2.5%–25% of pregnant women. Such discrepancy in the incidence of active rheumatic fever can be attributed to the inadequacy of the applied criteria. There is an opinion that depression of glucocorticoid secretion during pregnancy could activate the rheumatic process (Travyanko et al. 1981). At the same time, a more favorable course of pregnancy in women with rheumatic valvular heart disease and decreased number of complications due to a milder course of the disease and more effective therapy in the past decade have been reported (Szekely et al. 1973). However, in some cases metabolic and immunological shifts occurring in gestation activate the rheumatic process, namely rheumatic carditis which can lead to life-threatening cardiac decompensation. Active rheumatic carditis in some cases can be the cause of sudden death during labor or immediately after delivery. Recurrence of rheumatic endomyocarditis is most frequent in pregnant women with mitral stenosis, with mixed mitral valve disease and in combined valvular heart diseases including mitral stenosis (Chebotarev 1960). The rheumatic process is more frequently activated in the second rather than in the first half of gestation, with it sometimes recurring in the puerperium.

Recurrent rheumatic fever has an adverse effect on fetal development. Fetal hypoxia, intrauterine death, hypotrophy, premature delivery, postnatal asphyxia, and malformations are relatively often observed (Zakirov et al. 1979).

It is often difficult to detect a recurrence of the rheumatic process in gestation. Manifestations of acute articular inflammation are very rare. Subfebrile temperature can be caused either by pregnancy per se or by the presence of focal infection (cholecystitis, tonsilitis, etc.). Increased erythrocyte sedimentation rate and moderate leukocytosis can be also pregnancy induced. Sometimes during pregnancy leukocytosis can be substantial (up to 15000 cells/mm^3) due primarily to the increase in polymorphonuclear leukocytes (Quilligan 1982). Subfebrile temperature (in the absence of focal infection) in the prepregnancy period in women suffering from rheumatic fever suggests rheumatic fever recurrence. Pregnancy sometimes affects the findings of "rheumatic" tests; therefore, these tests should be complex and repetitive (Makolkin 1977). The techniques to determine the activity of the rheumatic process during pregnancy and in the puerperium, using cytological and immunofluorescent testing of colostrum and milk, have been suggested (Vanina et al. 1976, 1980). Recurrence of rheumatic carditis in a considerable number of pregnant women is associated with increased titers of antistreptohyaluronidase and antistreptolysine-0 (Zakirov et al. 1979). However, the increase in antistreptococcal antibody blood content can be caused by any streptococcal infection on the one hand, and, on the other hand, streptococcal infection manifestations are not always detected in a chronic rheumatic process. Immunological and biochemical findings should be considered only in the presence of clinical (even if equivocal) manifestations of the disease and rather marked shifts in these variables.

In suspected recurrence of rheumatic fever documented history data are essential. The patient's complaints of general weakness, easy fatigability, sweating, dyspnea, palpitation, and chest pains are nonspecific. The complaints of arthralgia and altered joint configuration are of more importance (however, rheumatic arthritis is rare in pregnancy, only occurring in constantly recurring rheumatic fever, which is life-threatening in pregnant women with severe myocardial and valvular lesions).

Rheumatic fever recurrence in pregnancy is usually not associated with a marked rise of body temperature, and subfebrile temperature is infrequent in normal pregnancy. Only when the body temperature is taken at 4-h intervals it is sometimes possible to detect its periodic elevation. Increased heart rate, more marked than in normal pregnancy, can sometimes be of certain diagnostic value. However, in the presence of valvular heart disease this finding reflects the onset of heart failure rather than recurrence of rheumatic fever.

Sometimes exacerbation of the rheumatic process is accompanied by a significant erythrocyte sedimentation rate increase, the increment being nonspecific in pregnancy. Complex biochemical testings (C-reactive protein, ceruloplasmin, oxyproline, α_2-globulins) and immunological findings are sometimes of relative value. It does not seem advisable for rheumatic fever diagnosis to determine the fibrinogen blood level, as it is always elevated in gestation.

Electrocardiographic changes are of certain value (P-Q interval lengthening, sometimes flattened, widened and notched P wave, QRS complex changes, modest ST segment, and T wave depression), but they are not always observed in recurrence of rheumatic fever.

In many cases, only a comprehensive assessment of history data, clinical, and laboratory findings makes it possible to reveal with a more or less high degree of certainty recurrence of rheumatic fever in pregnancy.

5 Acquired Valvular Heart Disease and Pregnancy

Valvular heart disease is encountered in 0.2%–4.7% of pregnant women (Jonáš 1960; Auinger 1967; Adams 1968; Etheridge 1969; Jorde and Morack 1970; Vanina 1971; Vasilenko 1972; Rush 1983). Such diverse data may be attributed to the absence of their standardized registration in pregnant women. Some authors make use of data from nonspecialized maternity centers (or units), others from hospitals (or units) dealing with nonobstetric pathology in pregnant women (not only cardiovascular). Some data were collected at the time when all heart diseases were considered as contraindications for pregnancy. Other data were collected in the past 2 decades, when the existing views were revised and pregnancy became permissible in many forms of valvular heart disease. Finally, the diagnostic accuracy and the proportion of women of childbearing age with cardiovascular diseases under medical care are of great importance for statistical findings. Thus, according to Vanina (1977a), 10% of women admitted to specialized units for pregnant women with cardiovascular diseases with the diagnosis of "valvular heart disease" reveal no disease, while in 27% of women valvular heart disease is first seen during pregnancy. The symptoms of mitral stenosis are first detected in gestation in 25% of affected patients (Sullivan and Ramanathan 1985).

Rheumatic valvular heart disease accounts for 75%–90% of all heart diseases occurring in pregnant women, congenital heart disease for 5%–15%, myocarditis, cardiomyopathies, coronary heart disease, and other heart diseases for not more than 4% (Etheridge 1969; Howitt 1971; Nesbitt and Abdul-Karim 1982; Deeg 1983; Perloff 1984). In many countries of the world the past decades have been characterized by a trend toward a reduction in the number of pregnant women with acquired valvular heart disease (though it is now allowed to retain pregnancy in an increasing number of cases) and a rise in the proportion of pregnant women with congenital heart disease. To some extent this might be related to a less severe course of the rheumatic process, advances in the treatment of rheumatic fever and prevention of rheumatic valvular heart disease, as well as timely diagnosis and successful surgical treatment of congenital heart disease, permitting increasing numbers of women with these anomalies to reach childbearing age. Each year the number of pregnant women who underwent cardiac surgery for congenital heart disease or acquired valvular heart disease prior to or during pregnancy is increasing. This may account for the fact that there are now fewer patients with severe valvular lesions among pregnant women with valvular heart disease. It should be also noted that in some developing countries (India, in particular) rheumatic (acute and chronic) heart disease is quite frequent among gravid females.

In the absence of heart failure many heart diseases (including some acquired valvular heart lesions) pose no threat during pregnancy. The degree of risk depends on the patient's age, the duration and severity of the disease, the nature of hemodynamic disturbances prior to and during pregnancy, the course of pregnancy (sometimes preeclampsia-eclampsia or extragenital and extracardiac diseases can give rise to heart failure), and, last but not least, on the accuracy and efficacy of cardiological care. Friedberg (1963) reported the dependence of maternal mortality on the severity of heart disease: in patients of functional class I and II (NYHA classification) it accounted for about 2% and in patients of class III and IV for about 16%. The highest mortality rate is observed in patients with atrial fibrillation. Vanina (1977b) reports that with adequate cardiological care the mortality rate in pregnant women with heart disease does not reach 1%. Pregnant women with heart failure, functional class III and IV, are at the highest risk, but adequate management of such patients (especially during labor) can end in the birth of normal children (Clark et al. 1985). Women with advanced heart failure seldom conceive; however, they sometimes do become pregnant in spite of long-standing amenorrhea caused by severe heart failure (Vanina 1977b).

There are a number of schemes measuring the risk of pregnancy and labor in women with valvular heart disease. Some of them are based on up to ten variables that are scored and summed up (Kaluzna 1977). A simple, but adequate, scheme was suggested by Vanina (1971). There exist four degrees of risk: I — pregnancy in women with valvular heart disease without heart failure or recurrence of rheumatic fever; II — pregnancy in women with valvular heart disease and manifestations of developing heart failure (dyspnea, tachycardia), rheumatic fever, active phase I; III — pregnancy in women with decompensated valvular heart disease and signs of predominant right ventricular failure, rheumatic fever, active phase II, recent atrial fibrillation, second stage of pulmonary hypertension; IV — pregnancy in women with decompensated valvular heart disease with left ventricular or total failure, rheumatic fever, active phase III, atrio- or cardiomegaly, long-standing atrial fibrillation with thromboembolic complications, third stage of pulmonary hypertension. Pregnancy is considered permissible in risk degrees I and II and contraindicated in degrees III and IV (in most cases these are patients with mitral stenosis).

If pregnancy occurs in women with valvular heart disease over 35 years of age or in patients with marked ventricular or/and atrial hypertrophy, paired premature beats and episodes of heart failure in the history of previous pregnancies it is associated with unfavorable prognosis for the mother and child.

It is often not easy to diagnose the early stages of heart failure in pregnancy. Marked dyspnea, its combination with coughing, stable moist rales at the lung bases, liver enlargement, pronounced engorgement of the neck veins, elevated venous pressure on the arms, and the development or increase of acrocyanosis should put physicians on their guard, as these are typical manifestations of heart failure.

5.1 Mitral Stenosis

Mitral stenosis is a predominant form of rheumatic valvular heart disease found in 75%–90% of pregnant women with acquired valvular heart disease (Vanina 1971; Krayenbühl and Siegenthaler 1974; Szekely and Snaith 1974; Deeg 1983; etc.). Hemodynamic shifts in mitral stenosis are due to impeded left ventricular filling (and left atrial emptying) arising as a result of scarring and fibrosis of the mitral leaflets and comissural fusion. Sufficient blood flow through the left atrioventricular orifice in such cases is possible only with an increase in left atrial pressure leading to pressure elevation in pulmonary veins and capillaries. With the pressure in pulmonary capillaries exceeding 30 mm Hg, fluid transudation from capillaries into alveoli begins, but patients with mitral stenosis and long-standing pulmonary congestion develop pulmonary edema at higher pulmonary capillary pressure. However, reduced serum protein level, frequent in pregnancy, can decrease the threshold of pulmonary capillary pressure above which pulmonary edema may develop. In long-standing mitral stenosis the initial reflectory narrowing is followed by sclerotic changes in pulmonary arterioles that lead to the elevation of pulmonary arteriolar pressure as the disease progresses, serving in this case as a protective mechanism against pulmonary edema. However, the mere presence of high pulmonary hypertension is associated with a serious risk for pregnant women.

Hemodynamic changes caused by pregnancy (especially the increase in BV and heart rate leading to the rise in transmitral gradient and left atrial pressure elevation), elevated pressure in pulmonary circulation and a trend toward a decrease in pulmonary vascular resistance (promoting higher blood filling in pulmonary circulation), dilution anemia, and the resulting overload of both ventricles constitute a potential threat for patients with mitral stenosis and beginning from the 12th–13th week of gestation can cause such serious complications as cardiac asthma, pulmonary edema, hemoptysis, severe atrial fibrillation, right ventricular failure, and arterial embolism. Atrial fibrillation considerably worsens a hemodynamic situation due both to missing of normal left atrial contractions and often to increased heart rate leading to the shortening of the diastole. As a result, even insignificant exercise may cause an abrupt fall of the cardiac output or the onset of acute pulmonary edema. The onset of right ventricular failure in pregnant women leads to the development of peripheral edema and partly to varicose vein dilatation. Chronic venous congestion, in its turn, increases the risk of pulmonary artery embolism. Subacute bacterial myocarditis is rare in mitral stenosis.

In patients with mitral stenosis, physiological adaptation to cardiac output fluctuations is limited. The increase in venous return can elevate pulmonary arterial pressure and can lead to the development of right ventricular failure, while physical effort and psychoemotional stress can cause syncope due to acute right ventricular failure and insufficient or no increase in cardiac output upon a drop in systemic vascular resistance (Perloff 1984). Heart failure in women suffering from mitral stenosis can first develop in the puerperium or even after the abortion. Pulmonary venous congestion and edema can arise any time during gestation. In patients with minimal or mild stenosis of the left atrioventricular orifice the risk of complications is not too high. The risk of pulmonary edema is the highest in weeks 20–30 of pregnancy, during labor, and immediately following delivery. Adequate functional state of the myocardium prior to or in early pregnancy will not guarantee the absence of pulmonary edema in the future, as anatomically moderate stenosis in conditions of altered hemodynamics peculiar to pregnancy can prove functionally severe. Sometimes pulmonary edema develops for the first time in asymptomatic pregnant women under 30 with insignificant heart enlargement and normal sinus rhythm (Szekely and Snaith 1974).

The development of pulmonary edema in late pregnancy drastically worsens the prognosis, causing a high mortality rate (almost 50% of the overall death rate in pregnant women with rheumatic valvular heart disease). A prompt development of refractory pulmonary edema in such cases is due to a considerable increase in BV and other pregnancy-induced hemodynamic shifts. The remote risk of death in these patients remains high within the 1st year after delivery. The long persistent disease leads to sclerosis of pulmonary artery branches; it is rarely complicated by pulmonary edema and more frequently with right ventricular failure.

Women with mitral stenosis, like patients with other valvular heart diseases, have complicated pregnancy and labor (threatened abortion, preeclampsia-eclampsia, premature labor, premature rupture of membranes, fetal hypoxia, and so forth), which in their turn have an adverse effect on the course of heart disease. Pregnant women with mitral stenosis more often than women with other valvular heart diseases have a narrow pelvis.

Clinical (and roentgenological) signs of mitral stenosis, like those of other valvular heart diseases, remain unchanged in gestation. The majority of patients have no typical rheumatic articular attacks in history. Patients with mild stenosis are usually asymptomatic especially in early pregnancy. Such typical complaints as dyspnea on exertion, weakness, and fatigue are not pathognomonic as they are quite common for normal pregnancy. Dyspnea at rest is of greater diagnostic value; however, it is mostly characteristic of marked stenosis. The patients can complain of coughing (dry or with scanty mucous sputum), hemoptysis, palpitation, irregular heart beat, nagging or stabbing chest pains unrelated to physical effort, nicturia, and peripheral edema.

The patients with mild stenosis have an unremarkable appearance. In marked stenosis the patients are characterized by cyanotic flushing and mild or pronounced cyanosis of lips and distal limb segments. If the valvular disease is formed in childhood, general physical underdevelopment is observed. Inspection can reveal increased precardiac or epigastric pulsation (the latter still increasing on inspiration) owing to right ventricular hypertrophy or sometimes pulsation in the third and fourth left intercostal spaces. In long-standing disease, especially starting in childhood, "cardiac hump" is observed — a diffuse bulge of the precardiac area of the anterior chest wall.

Palpation reveals enhanced cardiac impulse. Quite often the apical impulse is not palpated due to left ventricular displacement by the right ventricle. In marked stenosis there is a feeling of diastolic rumble ("cat's purring") over the heart apex, enhanced after physical exercise and in the left lateral position during postexpiratory apnea. Accentuated second heart sound over the pulmonary artery (especially during postexpiratory apnea) can be felt with the palm of the examining hand in the second left intercostal space.

Typical auscultatory markings are: accentuated first heart sound (the accentuation disappears in cusp fibrosis and calcinosis) and an opening snap detected over the heart apex immediately after the second heart sound, diastolic rumble — a low-frequency diastolic murmur occurring at different phases of diastole (protodiastolic, mesodiastolic, and presystolic) over the heart apex — and accentuated and sometimes split second heart sound over the pulmonary artery. In the left lateral position and in heart enlargement the point at which the diastolic rumble is auscultated is displaced laterally. Presystolic murmur disappears in atrial fibrillation. Some patients also show systolic murmur associated either with coexisting mitral regurgitation or with the development of relative tricuspid valve insufficiency (in considerable right ventribular enlargement). Auscultatory hallmarks of mitral stenosis are most apparent upon moderate physical exercise during postexpiratory apnea with the patient in the left lateral position.

During gestation, sometimes due to enhanced blood flow through the narrowed valve orifice, previously undetectable in insignificant orifice stenosis, murmurs peculiar to mitral stenosis could be auscultated (the same holds true for uncommon tricuspid valve orifice stenosis). As a result, mitral stenosis is sometimes first detected only during pregnancy often in its first half. At the same time in some cases pregnancy-induced attenuation of presystolic murmur usually heard in mitral stenosis over the heart apex and narrowing of the already small area of its auscultation can be revealed.

In mitral stenosis heart rhythm disturbances, atrial fibrillation in particular (usually a tachysystolic form), are quite frequent. A small weak pulse is often felt. Systolic BP lowering and certain diastolic pressure elevation resulting in decreased pulse pressure can be noted. Some patients, however, can develop arterial hypertension. Deterioration of right ventricular contractility leads to venous pressure increase. Circulation time is usually prolonged.

Roentgenological findings in patients with mild mitral stenosis show no significant changes of the heart shadow. As the degree of stenosis progresses, "heart waist" gradually disappears due to left atrial enlargement and then prominence of the left atrial appendage and pulmonary artery is noted in the posteroanterior projection. The right atrium is also enlarged and comprises the lower part of the convex segment of the right heart border. Lung hili are widened and the vascular pattern of the pulmonary fields is enhanced. On the lateral view the normal retrosternal clear space is obliterated by the enlarged right ventricle and right atrium.

In significant stenosis broad, sometimes notched P wave resulting from left atrial overload is recorded on the ECG in I and II leads (and sometimes in the chest leads), and right ventricular overload causes R wave increase in the right chest leads, S wave increase in the left chest leads, and ST segment depression and negative T wave in the right chest leads.

Phonocardiographic findings demonstrate high-amplitude first heart sound over the apex; the interval between the second heart sound and mitral valve opening snap shortens as stenosis progresses, while the interval between Q wave (ECG) and the first heart sound (phonocardiogram) increases, reaching 0.08–0.12 s (normally it is 0.04–0.06 s). In severe stenosis, fusion of the second heart sound and mitral valve opening snap is observed. Diastolic rumbles are also recorded, with protodiastolic murmur detected right after mitral valve opening snap and presystolic murmur usually followed immediately by the first heart sound.

Echocardiographic findings of mitral stenosis are: reduced rate of mitral valve anterior cusp closure, decreased excursion of the mitral valve and thickening of its cusps, abnormal direction of posterior cusp motion, and right ventricular dilatation (at advanced stages of the disease). Doppler ultrasound allows quantitative assessment of the valvular gradient.

Heart catheterization (revealing blood pressure elevation first in the left atrium and pulmonary artery, and then in the right ventricle and atrium) and angiocardiography are performed in pregnant women with valvular heart disease only when a possible surgical intervention is considered.

Severe mitral stenosis (when there is a combination of high pulmonary vascular resistance with low cardiac output, diastolic rumble over the apex can attenuate and even completely disappear; at the same time due to mitral valve calcification the opening snap and accentuation of the first heart sound over the apex can be absent) should be distinguished from the diseases associated with venous pulmonary hypertension and somewhat increased heart size, i.e., primary pulmonary hypertension and cor pulmonale. Differentiation between the diseases is necessary, as in the former case the necessity of surgical intervention can be discussed and in the two latter cases surgery in such a situation is out of the question. In such cases mitral valve stenosis is diagnosed by roentgenological findings of left atrial enlargement and mitral valve calcification. If necessary, pulmonary function is examined and heart catheterization is performed.

Precordial pulsation, accentuated first heart sound over the heart apex (sometimes diastolic murmur), and paroxysms of atrial fibrillation in patients with thyrotoxicosis can simulate the pattern of mitral stenosis. The correct diagnosis is facilitated by the detection of other symptoms and signs of thyrotoxicosis and biochemical examination of blood.

In rare cases, mitral stenosis should be differentiated from atrial septal defect (when the second heart sound splitting over the pulmonary artery is transmitted downwards to the left sternal edge and is considered mitral opening snap) or from mobile left atrial myxoma. In the latter case, auscultatory signs of mitral stenosis can be detected, sometimes persisting irrespective of body position changes. However, myxoma is often characterized by sudden appearance of mitral stenosis signs that can be accompanied by fits of unconsciousness (in complete obstruction of valvular orifice). Atrial myxoma can be accompanied by fever, anemia, and weight loss, with X-ray findings revealing only slight left atrial enlargement. Myxoma can be detected echocardiographically and angiocardiographically.

The following disorders can complicate mitral stenosis: hemoptysis, cardiac asthma, pulmonary edema, atrial fibrillation (or occasionally atrial flutter) often preceded by frequent atrial premature beats, paroxysmal atrial tachycardia, thromboembolism (ball thrombi in the left atrium, embolization of the cerebral, renal, spleen, and lower extremity arteries), phlebothrombosis of the lower extremities, often resulting in pulmonary infarction, symptoms of left recurrent nerve, left subclavian artery, and sometimes sympathetic nerve compression by a drastically enlarged left atrium.

According to Szekely and Snaith (1974), who in 1942–1971 examined 761 pregnant women (1102 pregnancies) with rheumatic valvular heart disease, out of 991 pregnancies in patients with mitral stenosis heart failure was observed in 23% of cases, with pulmonary congestion, pulmonary edema, and right ventricular failure recorded in 18.3%, 1.7%, and 2% of cases, respectively; in the past decade no cases of pulmonary edema and right ventricular failure were noted. Atrial fibrillation was observed in 7% of cases, paroxysmal atrial tachycardia in 3.4%, systemic embolism in 1.6% and pulmonary artery embolism in 1.8%. Pulmonary venous congestion was more frequent in women above 30 and in in multigravidas. Over the past 2 decades there has been a gradual decrease in the incidence and severity of mitral stenosis in pregnant women examined in antenatal clinics (Chesley 1980).

With the development of heart failure pregnant women with mitral valve stenosis show decreased stroke volume, cardiac output and heart work, increased (greater than in healthy women) BV, elevated pulmonary arterial pressure, and total systemic vascular resistance (Korenevskaya 1978), promoting the development of both pulmonary edema and right ventricular failure. The analysis of systolic time intervals in this case shows a considerable lengthening of left ventricular isometric contraction time and shortening of the ejection time resulting in the onset of cardiac hypodynamia syndrome. In some cases the enhanced right ventricular function can, in such conditions, contribute to greater congestion in the pulmonary vessels, leading to pulmonary edema. Thus, pulmonary congestion and edema are more frequent in pregnant than in nonpregnant patients with mitral stenosis.

Pulmonary edema in pregnant women can be caused by exertional sinus tachycardia and episodes of paroxysmal tachycardia, which are characterized by reduced blood flow through the mitral valve (due to the shortening of diastole) and secondary rapid elevation of the left atrial pressure.

5.2 Mitral Regurgitation

Mitral regurgitation is the second most frequent (6%–7%) type of acquired rheumatic valvular heart disease, detected in pregnancy. In rare cases it can be caused by systemic lupus erythematosus, bacterial endocarditis, scleroderma, and heart trauma. In the absence of pronounced regurgitation, heart rhythm disturbances, and heart failure, pregnancy does not have a detrimental effect on the coexisting valvular heart disease. Better adaptation of the cardiovascular system to pregnancy-induced rise in cardiac output and heart rate is observed in these patients, as compared with pregnant women with mitral stenosis. Pregnancy-induced reduction in total peripheral resistance facilitates left ventricular blood outflow, decreasing the degree of regurgitation and somewhat improving the patient's condition. The left ventricle copes fairly well with an increased blood volume; severe pulmonary hypertension is not usually typical of this pathology. With marked regurgitation, atrial fibrillation or flutter are associated with poor prognosis, as such patients usually have a dilated and impaired left ventricle. The risk of subacute bacterial endocarditis in mitral regurgitation is higher than in mitral stenosis. Acute enhancement of mitral regurgitation due to chordae tendineae rupture in rheumatic mitral valve incompetence almost always results from superimposed bacterial endocarditis (Reichek et al. 1973). However, during pregnancy acute mitral regurgitation resulting from spontaneous rupture of chordae tendineae can occur (Caves and Paneth 1972).

Hemodynamic shifts in mitral regurgitation are caused by incomplete closure of the deformed mitral leaflets resulting in backward blood flow into the left ventricle along with forward blood flow into the aorta. As a result, excessive blood volume is detected in the left atrium during systole and in the left ventricle during diastole. This leads to hypertrophy and dilatation of the left heart chambers. Distension of left atrial musculature by excessive blood volume makes its contractions more powerful. Due to left ventricular and left atrial enlargement, the mitral valve ring becomes distended and the degree of regurgitation increases. The powerful left ventricle compensates for intracardiac hemodynamic disturbances over a long period. Left atrial weakening is associated with a dramatic rise in intraatrial pressure. This leads to pulmonary vein engorgement causing venous pulmonary hypertension without severe elevation of pulmonary arterial pressure. At advanced stages of the disease, right heart overload develops, although less prominent than in mitral stenosis, but finally leading to congestion in systemic circulation.

In compensated mitral regurgitation the patients are asymptomatic in most cases. With impaired left ventricular contractility, the patients complain of palpitation, fatigability, exertional dyspnea (in heart failure the patients experience dyspnea at rest); however, such complaints are not infrequent in normal pregnancy as well. In pulmonary congestion the patients complain of dry (or with scanty sputum) coughing. Complaints of hemoptysis are much rarer than in mitral stenosis. In cases complicated by right ventricular failure the patients experience peripheral edema and pains in the right hypochondrium.

On inspection, no peculiarities are revealed long after the onset of the disease. At advanced stages, intensification of the apical impulses and their downward and lateral displacement are sometimes visually detected. If the disease developed in childhood "cardiac hump" may be observed to the left of the sternum. However, in women, except for those who are very thin, it is masked by the mammary gland. In marked heart failure acrocyanosis and cyanotic blush can be observed.

Palpation usually reveals intensified apical impulse in the fifth or sometimes in the sixth intercostal spaces laterally to the midclavicular line. With severe dilatation of the left ventricle, parasternal impulse can be palpated.

The main auscultatory hallmarks of mitral regurgitation are detected over the apex. The first heart sound is usually decreased in intensity, or remains normal; in rare cases it is accentuated, and rather often is masked by early systolic murmur. Moderately accentuated second heart sound is auscultated over the pulmonary artery (with the onset of right ventricular failure the accent may disappear). The second heart sound over the pulmonary artery can be split. In severe mitral regurgitation the third heart sound and early transient diastolic filling murmur are audible over the heart apex. Mitral valve opening snap is rarely heard.

A typical feature of mitral regurgitation is a loud systolic regurgitation murmur over the heart apex. It can be blowing or harsh. It is sometimes detected parasternally in the fourth left intercostal space. The murmur can be heard over part of the systole or more often over the whole systole (holosystolic murmur). Its duration and loudness usually correspond to the degree of mitral regurgitation. Auscultatory changes are better revealed with the patient in the left lateral position during postexpiratory apnea (and after moderate exercise). The murmur is usually well radiated to the axillar area, to the back, and often to the heart base.

It has been noted that the murmur typical of mitral regurgitation attenuates and even disappears in almost 50% of pregnant women with this form of valvular heart disease; the same is observed in pregnant women with mitral valve prolapse (Haas 1976). It is presumably due to pregnancy-induced reduction in total peripheral resistance, as with total peripheral resistance elevation (squatting, ephedrine injection) the sound reappears or intensifies. At the same time it should be borne in mind that the appearance of systolic murmur over the heart apex in normal pregnant women can be often mistaken for mitral regurgitation. To distinguish between murmurs of organic and functional mitral valve incompetence, one should consider the nature of the murmur (in the former case it is usually blowing, harsh, and coarse and in the latter case it is faint), its changes in response to physical exercise (in the former case, it increases in intensity and in the latter case it attenuates or even disappears), and its dependence on the body posture (in the former case it is equal in intensity in the upright and supine position, and in the latter case it is more intensive in the supine position, attenuating or even disappearing in the upright position). Finally, the functional murmur is less durable, with the first heart sound unchanged. However, sometimes it takes an X-ray examination to either confirm or discard the diagnosis of organic mitral regurgitation.

Heart rate and blood pressure remain unchanged in uncomplicated rheumatic mitral regurgitation, with atrial fibrillation occurring at advanced stages of the disease.

Radiological findings reveal moderate to considerable left ventricular and left atrial enlargement. Left ventricular enlargement — an obligatory sign of mitral regurgitation — is more easily detected in the left lateral or left oblique position with a barium-filled esophagus (the esophagus deviates along the high-radius arch). Sometimes additional left atrial enlargement is observed during systole. The symptoms of pulmonary hypertension and right ventricular failure are associated with right ventricular enlargement. In the absence of heart failure pulmonary vasculature patterns are normal. With the onset of heart failure, signs of pulmonary congestion are detected.

The electrocardiogram in marked mitral regurgitation shows signs of left atrial hypertrophy (widened, sometimes notched P wave in I and II leads and occasionally in chest leads); in less than half of the cases signs of left ventricular overload are observed (R wave and S wave amplitude increase in V_{5-6} leads and V_{1-2} leads, respectively, sometimes ST segment displacement and T wave changes including inversion in V_{5-6} and I leads). Right ventricular hypertrophy is associated with $R_{V_{1-2}}$ amplitude increase.

In pronounced mitral regurgitation the phonocardiogram reveals reduced amplitude of the first heart sound. It can be masked by systolic murmur. The third heart sound can be recorded over the heart apex not earlier than 0.12 s after the second heart sound. Systolic murmur is recorded right after or simultaneously with the first heart sound, and can last throughout the whole systole, with its amplitude reducing in late systole. The murmur amplitude usually corresponds to the degree of valvular incompetence.

Echocardiography reveals enlargement of anteroposterior left atrial (at advanced stages also left ventricular) size and increased amplitude of ventricular septal contractions. Thickening of mitral valve cusps can be detected. At advanced stages of the disease the right ventricular cavity is well visualized. Doppler ultrasound technique permits the detection and quantitative assessment of mitral regurgitation.

In the absence of history data and documented findings indicative of previous rheumatic fever the need for differential diagnosis often arises as systolic murmur over the heart apex can be audible not only in organic mitral regurgitation and in normal pregnancy (as a manifestation of functional valvular incompetence and hemodynamics shifts) but also in a number of other diseases. It is easy to distinguish systolic murmur caused by anemia or thyrotoxicosis (there are usually other typical signs of the diseases). If the murmurs are functional there are no roentgenological findings of left atrial or ventricular enlargement, electrocardiographic signs of left heart overload, or echocardiographic signs of organic mitral valve lesions. Coarse systolic murmur can be auscultated in aortic valvular stenosis and ventricular septal defect; however, in these cases the murmur is usually the loudest not over the heart apex but parasternally in the second right and the fourth left intercostal spaces respectively. In the presence of aortic stenosis it is radiated into the carotids and to the apex, but not the axillary area. Amylnitrite inhalation intensifies the murmur in patients with aortic stenosis and attenuates it in patients with mitral regurgitation, while intravenous phenylephrine injection has an opposite effect on the murmur intensity. Finally, the murmur intensity typical of mitral regurgitation remains unchanged after premature beats. In addition, there are other symptoms typical of aortic stenosis and ventricular septal defect. In rare cases, to differentiate between mitral regurgitation and aortic stenosis or ventricular septal defect, heart catheterization or angiocardiography are performed (in pregnancy only when surgical intervention is considered). It is difficult to differentiate between rheumatic and nonrheumatic mitral regurgitation in the absence of sufficient history data. The question is of utmost importance, as in the former case medical therapy to prevent rheumatic fever recurrence is necessary. The combination of mitral regurgitation with mitral stenosis or with other valve damage indicates the rheumatic origin of the disease. Spontaneous rupture of the chordae tendinaea is accompanied by sudden appearance of valvular incompetence signs in the absence of left heart chamber enlargement (or in the presence of insignificant enlargement). Frequently, the fourth heart sound is auscultated after the third heart sound; the sinus rhythm remains undisturbed. In some cases rheumatic mitral regurgitation should be differentiated from regurgitation caused by mitral valve prolapse (the murmur is mostly late), hypertrophic cardiomyopathy (idiopathic hypertrophic subaortic stenosis), and Marfan's syndrome and the Enlers-Danlos syndrome. Though all these diseases have their characteristic signs sometimes it is only angiocardiographically that all the diagnostic problems can be solved (Kremkau et al. 1973).

The complications in mitral regurgitation are almost the same as in mitral stenosis. However, their frequency is different. Thus, the incidence of pulmonary edema is eight times lower in mitral regurgitation (though the rise in the cardiac output in pregnancy increases in regurgitation), hemoptysis is half as frequent, and subacute bacterial endocarditis complicates mitral regurgitation more often than mitral stenosis (Silber and Katz 1975). According to Szekely and Snaith (1974), pregnant women with mitral regurgitation develop heart failure in 5.5% of cases. In the majority of cases pulmonary congestion (but not edema) is observed. Atrial fibrillation, paroxysmal atrial tachycardia, pulmonary thromboembolism, and bacterial endocarditis develop in 4.2%, 5.5%, 2.9%, and 8.5% of cases, respectively. It should be noted that in recent years the incidence of bacterial endocarditis became much lower in pregnant women due to preventive therapy with antibiotics.

5.3 Aortic Regurgitation

Aortic valvular disease is less frequently observed in pregnancy (in 0.75%–5% of pregnant women with acquired valvular heart disease) than mitral valvular disease; however, the risk of acute heart failure in pregnant women with aortic valvular disease is extremely high. Some signs of heart failure are detected in 85% of such pregnant women (Vitushkina and Popova 1977). The onset of heart failure during pregnancy or labor in women with aortic valvular disease renders the disease refractory to therapy and causes the patients' condition to deteriorate rapidly. Aortic valvular disease may combine with other valve lesions (e.g., mitral).

Aortic regurgitation is more frequent than valvular aortic stenosis and in the majority of cases is of rheumatic origin. Sometimes regurgitation is caused by rheumatoid arthritis, bacterial endocarditis, syphilis, Marfan's syndrome, blunt chest trauma, or aortic valve prolapse (usually combined with mitral valve prolapse). Aortic regurgitation is caused by scarring, shortening, retraction, and rigidity of the leaflets.

Hemodynamic shifts in this valvular disease are caused by blood regurgitation from the aorta to the left ventricle during diastole due to incomplete closure of the valvular leaflets. The degree of regurgitation is determined by the magnitude of diastolic aperture of the valvular orifice. Owing to a high diastolic pressure gradient between the aorta and the left ventricle, blood reflux from the aorta will be great if the diastolic valvular aperture accounts for only one-sixth of the normal valvular orifice area during systole. At a higher heart rate, regurgitation volume may be smaller due to the shortening of diastole. Reversed blood flow into the left ventricle leads to its dilatation and (later) hypertrophy; however, end-diastolic left ventricular pressure remains normal for a long while due to the increased ventricular muscle compliance and rises only (like end-diastolic left atrial pressure) with the onset of heart failure. Systolic output in aortic regurgitation is usually highly elevated, with compensatory reduction in aortic resistance and total peripheral resistance. In high-degree left ventricular dilatation distension of the mitral valve tendinous ring and secondary mitral incompetence can develop. Commonly this is promptly followed by hyperfunction and then left atrial and right ventricular hypertrophy and possibly right ventricular failure. In pregnancy a rise in BV increases left ventricular load, and, on the other hand, a heart rate increase in pregnant women leads to the shortening of diastole and finally to the decrease of regurgitation volume. This is also promoted by additional pregnancy-induced reduction in the total peripheral resistance.

The patients with hemodynamically significant aortic regurgitation are usually asymptomatic for many years. With progression of the disease, they develop feelings of increased force of heart contractions and beats against the chest wall (most intensive in the left lateral position), feelings of intensified pulsation of the carotids and other major peripheral arteries, dizziness, and predisposition to syncope (due to insufficient brain blood supply), and attacks of chest pain (due to reduced coronary blood flow resulting from marked reduction in diastolic pressure). Dyspnea after moderate physical exercise usually marks the termination of a relatively benign period. Later on, dyspnea at rest and, with the development of right ventricular failure, pains in the right hypochondrium and edema ensue.

The inspection of patients with marked aortic regurgitation reveals skin pallor, visible pulsation of carotids, temporal, and other superficial peripheral arteries, pulse-synchronized head noddings, alternate reddening and blanching of the nail bed, and alternate narrowing and widening of eye pupils with every heart beat. In pronounced aortic regurgitation increased diffuse apical impuls is usually displaced laterally and inferiorly (to the sixth left intercostal space). Sometimes rhythmic retraction and bulging of intercostal tissues adjacent to the apical impulse area are noted. Chest palpation reveals the "lifting" apical impulse. Pulsation of the aortic arch and abdominal part of the aorta is palpated in the jugular pit and epigastral area, respectively.

Auscultation in severe regurgitation reveals attenuated first and second heart sounds over the apex and at the heart base, respectively. Faint blowing diastolic murmur of decreasing intensity in the third and fourth left intercostal spaces (usually in rheumatic valvular heart disease) and in the second right intercostal space (more often in nonrheumatic valvular heart disease) are characteristic features of aortic regurgitation. The murmur is radiated to the heart apex. The duration and intensity of the murmur in most cases correlates with the pressure gradient between the aorta and the left ventricle. In some cases (more often in nonrheumatic valvular heart disease) the sound has a "musical" pitch. In the second right intercostal space systolic murmur is often audible which is always caused by the relative narrowing of the valvular orifice rather than by organic stenosis: the murmur is radiated to the neck vessels. Finally, in this heart valvular disease presystolic rumble (Flint's murmur) can be asucultated over the heart apex. It is caused by relative stenosis of the left atrioventricular orifice in late diastole due to anterior mitral cusp lifting by the regurgitating blood flow. The third heart sound (left ventricular filling sound) can be also heard over the apex. At early stages the murmur is better heard with the patient in the sitting-stooping position or the knee-elbow position. Typical heart murmurs can attenuate and in rare cases even disappear (at early stages of the disease) during pregnancy in women with aortic (as well as with mitral) regurgitation.

Radial artery pulse in aortic regurgitation is characterized by a rapid and marked rise and rapid collapse. Systolic BP is elevated (sometimes substantially) and diastolic pressure is lowered (and is sometimes undetectable by auscultatory method), while pulse pressure increases. Systolic pressure on the legs can exceed systolic pressure on the arms by 20–60 mmHg. Applying mild pressure with a stethoscope one can detect double (systolic and diastolic) bruit over the carotid or femoral arteries. Venous pressure in the absence of heart failure remains virtually unchanged.

Roentgenological findings in mild and even moderate aortic regurgitation reveal no essential changes of the heart shadow. In severe valvular incompetence the heart shadow is enlarged due to left ventricular dilatation. The heart apex shadow may be elongated posteriorly and inferiorly. The shadow of the ascending aorta is sometimes widened and its intensified pulsation is visible. Heart failure is accompanied by pulmonary congestion.

The electrocardiogram in advanced aortic regurgitation is changed. $R_{V_{5-6}}$ and $S_{V_{1-2}}$ amplitudes are increased; tall, peaked T waves and deep Q waves are recorded in V_{4-6} leads. Later the signs of left atrial overload can appear. Heart rhythm disturbances are rare.

Phonocardiography reveals the same changes in the heart sounds and the same murmurs as auscultation. However, sometimes at the early stages of the disease high-frequency murmurs detected by auscultation are recorded poorly or not at all on the phonocardiogram.

Echocardiography reveals an increase in anteroposterior left ventricular dimensions and increased amplitude of ventricular septal and left ventricular free wall contractions. Widening of the aortic root, regurgitation-induced mitral valve anterior cusp oscillations, and sometimes premature mitral valve closure are observed. The degree of regurgitation can be quantitatively assessed by Doppler echocardiography.

Heart catheterization and angiocardiography are performed in pregnancy only when surgical intervention is considered necessary.

In aortic regurgitation the compensatory period usually lasts for many years; however, once heart failure develops it becomes extremely difficult or even impossible to restore compensation. Therefore, pregnancy-induced hemodynamic shifts combined with physical and psychoemotional stress in women who have long suffered from this form of valvular disease are associated with a great risk and may irreversibly damage an already unstable compensation. First of all, dyspnea on mild exertion and at rest will develop; this may be followed by cardiac asthma and pulmonary edema. Szekely and Snaith (1974) reported that heart failure is detected in 7% of pregnant women with aortic regurgitation (all these patients had pulmonary edema).

Aortic regurgitation can combine with mitral regurgitation, which is hemodynamically manifested in reduced cardiac output. The combination of these two defects can be detected during auscultation, although the degree of severity of each defect is impossible to assess clinically, as the symptoms and signs of one mask those of the other. In such cases if the woman insists upon continuing the pregnancy the need for heart catheterization and angiocardiography arises to assess the expediency and feasibility of cardiac surgery.

5.4 Aortic Stenosis

Aortic ostium stenosis can be valvular (due to valvular commissural fusion), subvalvular (due to fibrous narrowing below the valves or pronounced hypertrophy of the left ventricular outflow pathways), and supravalvular. The latter two forms are usually considered congenital, with the etiological role of genetic factors not excluded. In women of childbearing age valvular aortic stenosis is mostly of rheumatic origin, and, in some cases, can be caused by bacterial endocarditis. It is often combined with aortic regurgitation and/or rheumatic mitral valvular disease.

Isolated or predominant rheumatic aortic valvular stenosis is relatively infrequent in pregnant women (1%–2% of the total number of patients with acquired valvular heart disease). Due to commissural fusion and thickening and fibrous degeneration of the valvular cusps, this form of the defect is characterized by a peculiar dome-shaped diaphragm with a small-diameter orifice. The damaged valve is often calcified. As a result, blood flow from the left ventricle into the aorta is hindered. The obstruction becomes hemodynamically significant if the aortic orifice area decreases by 50%; a 75% reduction decreases the cardiac output. Compensatory mechanisms, ensuring sufficient cardiac output in this form of valvular heart disease, are left ventricular systolic pressure elevation and prolongation of its systole, both events associated with left ventricular hypertrophy (unlike aortic regurgitation, left ventricular dilatation in aortic stenosis occurs only in heart failure). In heart failure end-diastolic left ventricular pressure elevation is followed by a rise in left atrial and pulmonary venous pressure. At terminal stages right ventricular failure can develop. In pregnant women with this valvular heart disease BV and cardiac output increase is accompanied by left ventricular systolic pressure elevation, possibly increasing the likelihood of heart failure development. Coronary perfusion in aortic stenosis is significantly decreased. A drop in BP owing to pregnancy-induced decrease in peripheral vascular resistance can, to a great extent, worsen coronary perfusion (Sullivan and Ramanathan 1985).

In rheumatic aortic valvular stenosis, as in aortic regurgitation, the patients remain asymptomatic for a long period and tolerate significant physical activity well. If cardiac output drops below the normal level, dyspnea (initially only on exertion), dizziness, syncope, and chest pain caused by inadequate cerebral and coronary blood flow appear. It should be noted that the presence of two or three of these symptoms considerably worsens the prognosis. With the onset of left or right ventricular failure the patients voice complaints typical of these complications.

On inspection, skin pallor (in pronounced stenosis) and acrocyanosis (in heart failure) are observed.

Palpation of the precardiac area in patients with pronounced aortic stenosis reveals an apical impulse of increased intensity and prolonged duration, displaced laterally (slightly — in the stage of compensation or considerably — in decompensation) and downward (usually in decompensation). Palpation in the second right intercostal space and the third and fourth left intercostal spaces as well as in the jugular pit and carotid areas reveals a systolic thrill, increasing in the supine position during postexpiratory apnea and vanishing with the onset of heart failure.

In severe stenosis the first heart sound is usually present and is sometimes split, the second heart sound being either normal or faint. Coarse mesosystolic murmur (reaching its maximum at midsystole) is a specific feature of the disease. It is well audible in the second right intercostal space and the third and fourth left intercostal spaces and radiates into the carotids (sometimes also into the interscapular area). The murmur also radiates to the apex (an ejection click can be also heard). As in other valvular heart diseases, the murmur is better heard with the patient in the supine position during postexpiratory apnea. In significant stenosis systolic BP and pulse pressure are lowered. Radial artery pulse is of small amplitude, gradually sloping up: bradycardia is quite frequent. Venous pressure and circulation time in the state of compensation are normal.

X-rays of severe stenosis reveal different degrees of ventricular enlargement (in heart failure also left atrial and right ventricular enlargement), sometimes aortic valvular calcification, and poststenotic dilatation of the ascending aorta.

The electrocardiographic findings make it possible to assess the degree of stenosis and to determine the presence of coronary insufficiency and episodes of atrioventricular and intraventricular conduction disturbances (or sometimes persistent conduction disturbances). In mild to moderate aortic stenosis the electrocardiogram can be normal. As left ventricular hypertrophy develops, $R_{V_{5-6}}$ and $S_{V_{1-2}}$ wave amplitude increases and T wave amplitude decreases (they can become diphasic or even negative) in I lead and leads V_{9-6}; ST segment depression is recorded in the same leads.

Phonocardiogram registers typical spindle-shaped systolic murmur oscillations occurring soon after the first heart sound and ceasing in protodiastole. The aortic component of the second heart sound is of lower intensity or altogether absent, while its pulmonary component (recorded in the second left intercostal space) is usually present.

Echocardiographic findings demonstrate thickening, calcification, and decreased mobility of aortic valve cusps, as well as left ventricular wall thickening. At advanced stages of the disease an increase in anteroposterior left ventricular dimensions is noted. Doppler ultrasound technique makes it possible to determine the valvular gradient. Echocardiographic criteria permit timely detection of the initial manifestations of heart failure (Titchenko 1986).

In dubious cases differential diagnosis with hypertrophic obstructive cardiomyopathy, coarctation of the aorta, pulmonary artery stenosis, atrial septal defect, and congenital subvalvular and supravalvular aortic stenosis is performed. When diagnosis is unclear or when the necessity and feasibility of surgical intervention is considered, heart catheterization and angiography are performed.

The following complications are observed: bacterial endocarditis, sudden death [in 5%–18% of patients with severe aortic stenosis, sometimes asymptomatic, according to Shaffer and Silber (1975)] probably caused by acute conduction disturbances or acute coronary insufficiency; atrioventricular and intraventricular conduction disorders; heart failure; and angina pectoris.

The outcomes of this valvular heart disease in pregnant women may be unfavorable: maternal mortality — 17%, fetal mortality — 32%, death during therapeutic abortion — 40% (Arias and Pineda 1978).

Szekely and Snaith (1974) have not observed bacterial endocarditis and systemic embolism in pregnant women with this valvular heart disease; heart failure developed in 35% of cases (17% of these patients had pulmonary edema, and 83% had pulmonary congestion); attacks of angina pectoris or unconsciousness were noted in 14.5% of cases.

5.5 Tricuspid Regurgitation

Rheumatic tricupid valve lesions are rather frequently found during postmortem examinations, although the degree of valve alterations is rarely hemodynamically significant. Tricuspid regurgitation and tricuspid stenosis are predominant in females. Tricuspid regurgitation can be both organic and functional (in the former case there are morphological alterations of valvular cusps, usually less marked than mitral valve lesions; in the latter case valvular cusps are unchanged, with only their tendinous ring or papillary muscles distended due to pronounced right ventricular dilatation). Tricuspid regurgitation is commonly of rheumatic origin; it infrequently results from subacute bacterial endocarditis, some congenital heart anomalies, and rarely from endomyocardial fibroelastosis or blunt chest trauma. In rheumatic fever this valvular disease is often associated with mitral (sometimes aortic) valve lesions. Functional tricuspid regurgitation is most frequent in severe pulmonary hypertension (terminal stage of mitral stenosis, cor pulmonale).

Hemodynamic shifts in this defect are caused by blood regurgitation during systole from the right ventricle into the right atrium, inducing their dilation. Then the regurgitating blood together with the blood flowing from the caval veins fills the right ventricle, inducing right ventricular pressure elevation, ventricular dilatation, and hypertrophy. In the presence of pulmonary hypertension, blood outflow from the right ventricle is impeded, further complicating the situation. The thin right atrial wall has limited compensatory capacity, and therefore blood congestion and pressure elevation are transmitted to caval veins. As pregnancy is also characterized by a rise in right ventricular pressure and venous pressure on the legs, all these shifts put together seem prognostically unfavorable.

The patients complain of weakness rather than of dyspnea (dyspnea is present in predominant combined mitral stenosis); they experience pain in the right hypochondrium and lack of appetite.

Inspection reveals acrocyanosis, neck vein distension, and their systolic pulsation (positive venous pulse); at advanced stages ascitis and peripheral edema can be observed. In severe tricuspid regurgitation pulsation of the right ventricle and liver is visible in the epigastral area and right hipochondrium, respectively; in less marked regurgitation the pulsation can be palpated. Palpation usually detects cardiac impulse, while apical impulse is undetectable. The heart is enlarged due to right atrial dilation, while in combined valvular heart disease the heart is sometimes enlarged leftwards. Percussion and palpation reveal liver enlargement (except for cases of congestive liver cirrhosis).

Crescendo blowing murmur lasting throughout the whole systole and best heard to the left of the xiphoid process base or sometimes in the fifth or fourth right intercostal spaces is a specific feature of tricuspid regurgitation. Unlike murmurs peculiar to rheumatic lesions of other valves, tricuspid regurgitation murmur is intensified during inspiration (and not expiration). The murmur radiates to the heart apex and almost never to the axillary area. In traumatic tricuspid regurgitation the murmur can be absent or is faint and short-term. In the presence of other forms of valvular heart disease peculiar murmurs and heart sound alterations are auscultated; however, with the onset of tricuspid regurgitation the second heart sound accentuation over the pulmonary artery can disappear. Auscultation in most cases also reveals atrial fibrillation.

Blood pressure remains virtually unchanged. Venous pressure rises considerably, and circulation time increases.

Roentgenological findings reveal right ventricular and right atrial enlargement. Other changes depend on the type of valvular heart disease combined with tricuspid regurgitation and the severity of pulmonary hypertension.

The electrocardiogram in isolated tricuspid regurgitation exhibits patterns of right atrial hypertrophy: tall, peaked $P_{II, III}$ and $P_{aVF, V_{1-2}}$ waves. However, the electrocardiographic changes typical of other concomitant valvular heart defects influence the general pattern of tricuspid regurgitation. Atrial fibrillation is typical.

The phonocardiogram records systolic murmur over tricuspid valve projection, intensified upon inspiration.

Echocardiography shows diminished or paradoxical movement of the interventricular septum, sometimes systolic prolapse of the tricuspid valve cusps and distended right ventricular cavity.

In some cases it becomes necessary to differentiate between isolated tricuspid regurgitation, adhesive pericarditis, which is quite easy, and right atrial tumor (with the help of angiocardiography).

5.6 Tricuspid Stenosis

Tricuspid stenosis is a rare pathology observed almost exclusively in women. Tricuspid rheumatic stenosis is usually combined with mitral (sometimes also aortic) valve lesions and is seldom an isolated valvular heart defect. Tricuspid stenosis may be found in patients with systemic lupus erythematosus, endomyocardial fibroelastosis, or carcinoid syndrome.

Hemodynamic shifts in tricuspid stenosis are caused by impeded right ventricular blood filling due to partial cusp fusion, thickening, and wrinkling. This is practically always accompanied by different degrees of valvular regurgitation, in part, probably, because the right atrioventricular orifice is the largest. The right atrium, lacking a sufficiently potent muscle, is rapidly hypertrophied and dilated; in severe stenosis a giant right atrium can be observed. With concomitant mitral stenosis, the right ventricle can be also hypertrophied. In tricuspid stenosis the right atrial-right ventricular pressure gradient is lower than the left atrial-left ventricular gradient in mitral stenosis; however, the caval veins are unprotected by the valves, and elevated right atrial pressure increases systemic venous pressure, aggravating varicose vein dilatation on the legs and in the pelvis and promoting the development of peripheral edema. Increased heart rate and augmented cardiac output (hemodynamic shifts that can also be observed in pregnancy) induce a rise in venous return and increase the pressure gradient, thereby complicating the situation. In certain cases (severe stenosis) insufficient right (and left) ventricular blood filling leads to cardiac output reduction, which can constitute a certain threat during exertion, including labor. The pressure gradient increases during inspiration and decreases during expiration due to changes in venous return. In tricuspid stenosis combined with mitral stenosis pulmonary and left atrial pressure is not as high as in isolated mitral stenosis. However, tricuspid stenosis is characterized by early systemic congestion.

The patients complain of dyspnea (caused by hypoxemia and in the case of associated mitral stenosis, partly related to pulmonary congestion), weakness, pain in the right hypochondrium, dyspepsia, and sometimes palpitation.

Inspection reveals cyanosis with a yellowish tint, neck vein distention (no positive venous pulse is observed in the absence of tricuspid regurgitation), and sometimes ascitis and leg edema.

The apical impulse is hard to palpate, while enlarged and painful liver is well palpated. Sometimes diastolic thrill is detected at the lower left sternal border.

Auscultation reveals either unaltered or split and accentuated first heart sound over tricuspid valve projection; tricuspid valve opening snap can also be heard. The second heart sound is faint in the second left intercostal space. A specific feature of the disease is soft or loud diastolic murmur with presystolic amplification (sometimes only presystolic murmur) heard in the fourth and fifth left intercostal spaces and/or over the xiphoid process. In some cases the murmur can radiate to the heart apex and can be mistaken for mitral stenosis murmur. In such cases it should be recognized that in mitral stenosis the murmur does not radiate to the xiphoid process. In addition, in mitral stenosis the murmur intensifies during expiration, while in tricuspid stenosis the murmur intensification takes place during inspiration (the latter observation does not hold true in the case of pronounced heart failure). In the same way, one can distinguish between mitral and tricuspid valve opening snap. In the presence of concomitant tricuspid regurgitation holosystolic murmur of varying intensity is heard. In coexisting mitral or aortic valve lesions the corresponding alterations of heart sounds and murmurs are observed. Atrial fibrillation can be revealed in tricuspid stenosis.

Blood pressure is sometimes lowered due to cardiac output decrease. Systemic venous pressure is considerably elevated. Circulation time is prolonged.

X-rays reveal considerable right atrial enlargement. Isolated tricuspid stenosis is not associated with tricuspid valve calcification or symptoms of lung congestion. In combined valvular heart disease corresponding roentgenological signs appear.

The electrocardiogram exhibits patterns of marked right atrial hypertrophy and dilatation: tall, peaked $P_{II, III, aVF, V_{1-2}}$ waves and P-R interval prolongation. The characteristic patterns become obscure with the onset of atrial fibrillation frequent in this disease.

Phonocardiogram (better during inspiration) records spindle-shaped presystolic murmur and sometimes also tricuspid valve opening snap in the fifth left intercostal space. In coexisting valvular regurgitation systolic murmur is registered.

The echocardiogram (if the tricuspid valve is adequately located) demonstrates tricuspid valve changes identical to mitral valve changes in mitral stenosis.

Since in the early stages clinical manifestations of tricuspid stenosis are poorly expressed and are sometimes confused with symptoms of mitral stenosis, heart catheterization and angiocardiography are sometimes necessary. The detection of an uncommon tricuspid stenosis associated with mitral stenosis quite frequent in pregnancy is of great importance, especially when surgical correction of mitral valve during pregnancy is planned. Undetected and persistent tricuspid stenosis can make surgery ineffective.

The most frequent complication of tricuspid stenosis is congestive liver cirrhosis.

5.7 Acquired Lesions of the Pulmonic Valve

Rheumatic pulmonic valve disease is seldom diagnosed clinically but is more often found during postmortem examination. It is always combined with other valvular lesions. In rheumatic valvular pulmonic stenosis a typical systolic murmur can be heard in the second left intercostal space; other symptoms are usually masked by manifestations of other coexisting valvular heart defects. Valvular pulmonic stenosis is more often congenital.

Severe pulmonary hypertension in patients with mitral stenosis can be accompanied by functional pulmonic valve incompetence. In this case short blowing diastolic murmur is heard in the second left intercostal space. However, symptoms of pulmonary hypertension should be present, as the murmur in some cases can radiate from the third and fourth intercostal spaces and can be caused by aortic regurgitation.

5.8 Rheumatic Combined Valvular Heart Disease

Rheumatic combined valvular heart disease is quite frequent. Its diagnosis is complicated by the fact that hemodynamic shifts and signs typical of an individual valvular defect are not simply summed up but sometimes hinder the manifestation of some hemodynamic shifts and clinical signs characteristic of each form. Commonly, one of the two (or more) valvular lesions is predominant, its clinical and laboratory findings prevailing. The detection of a coexisting valvular heart disease in pregnant women is an important task, as it can play an essential role when the decision is to be made on the possibility to retain pregnancy or the surgical correction of the valvular defect. As the examination of such patients is complicated, often requiring heart catheterization and angiocardiography, pregnant women with suspected combined valvular heart disease should be examined in specialized cardiological or cardio-surgical units or hospitals.

6 Congenital Heart Disease and Pregnancy

6.1 Congenital Cardiovascular Anomalies

Accurate diagnosis and treatment of congenital heart disease have become possible only in the past 30–40 years owing to the improvement of diagnostic techniques (cardiac catheterization with manometry, angiography, and angiocardiography, echocardiography, etc.) and the development of surgical methods for radical and palliative correction of the heart and great vessel anomalies. For quite a long period all the congenital forms of heart disease were divided into two groups: "cyanotic" and "acyanotic". At present about 50 forms of congenital heart and great vessel disease are known, some of them quite rare, others encountered mainly in infancy and early childhood (the patients die because they are not treated surgically in good time or because effective methods of surgical correction of such anomalies have not been developed), and some diagnosed relatively often in women of childbearing age. This third group of congenital heart diseases will be reviewed in this chapter. Investigations on adult patients have found that atrial septal defect and patent ductus arteriosus predominate in females while ventricular septal defect occurs with equal frequency in males and females. And although pulmonic valve stenosis, tetralogy of Fallot, and coarctation of the aorta predominate in males, these congenital heart diseases can also be found in pregnant women.

Congenital heart disease can in some cases be transmitted by genetic factors or mediated by environmental factors. It has been established (Lequime et al. 1970) that the incidence of congenital heart disease in children of healthy mothers does not exceed 0.5%. The incidence of the disease in siblings of patients suffering from congenital heart disease is 1.5%–3% (Campbell 1965), which is at least three times higher than the incidence in the population. Almost the same incidence (2.6%–3.7%) is noted in children who have at least one parent with atrial or ventricular septal defect (Nora et al. 1969). It may increase considerably if both parents suffer from congenital heart disease. According to some new data, 16.1% of 372 children born to 233 mothers with congenital heart disease (about 50% of them had cardiac surgery before pregnancy) also suffered from congenital heart disease. The defect in 35 of 60 children was concordant with mother's cardiovascular anomalies; the majority of children born to mothers with ventricular septal defect and patent ductus arteriosus had, like their mothers, left-to-right shunt (Whittemore et al. 1982). In most cases congenital heart disease is sporadic, although some forms of the disease, more often than others, are hereditary. This holds true in the case of patent ductus arteriosus, atrial septal defect, idiopathic hypertrophic subaortic stenosis (more often considered as cardiomyopathy), dextrocardia, familial congenital complete atrioventricular block, Wolff-

Parkinson-White syndrome, Jervell and Lange-Nielsen syndrome, and supravalvular aortic stenosis. Mothers with congenital heart disease can have children with multiple cardiovascular anomalies (Lieber et al. 1985).

Environmental factors also play an important role in the development of congenital heart disease. Rubella in the first 2–3 months of pregnancy can cause failure of ductus arteriosus closure, and can give rise to atrial septal defect, isolated pulmonary artery stenosis, and tetralogy of Fallot. Herpes virus infection in the first months of gestation also increases the risk of tetralogy of Fallot development in the fetus. There are data on the positive correlation between seasonal outbreaks of respiratory infectious diseases and increased incidence of congenital heart disease in infants, born 8–9 months after infectious outbreaks (Lequime et al. 1970). The teratogenic effect of ionizing radiation and numerous chemical compounds, including drugs, is well known. The use of thalidomide in the first weeks of gestation caused not only limb malformations (phocomelia) but also septal anomalies. Children with patent ductus arteriosus and atrial and ventricular septal defect are much more often born to women who live in high-altitude areas.

Some noncardiac diseases are also of importance. Malformations are detected more often than usual in children of mothers suffering from diabetes mellitus and prediabetes.

Modern diagnostic techniques (including functional ones) make it possible not only to determine accurately the form and severity of congenital heart disease but also to assess adaptive capacity of the myocardium. This allowed some young women suffering from congenital heart disease to conceive, whereas earlier, pregnancy in such cases was considered a great risk to life. Due to the above, and also thanks to the decrease in the incidence of rheumatic heart disease in developed countries, the number and relative prevalence of pregnant women with congenital heart disease has considerably increased. Thus, in Newcastle (Great Britain) the ratio of pregnant women with acquired valvular heart disease to pregnant women with congenital heart disease was 20:1 in 1942–1951, and only 3:1 in 1962–1971 (Szekely and Snaith 1974), while in Leicester it was 1:3 in 1974–1982 (MacNab and Macafee 1985). On the other hand, in developed countries the number of patients with congenital heart disease who have been successfully operated on in childhood is increasing; successful operations are performed in women of childbearing age suffering from acquired heart disease. Therefore, there has appeared a new population of pregnant women — postoperative cardiac patients. Thus, according to different data, the incidence of congenital heart disease in pregnant women ranges from 0.5% to 10% of all heart diseases found in them. Atrial septal defect, patent ductus arteriosus, and ventricular septal defect are most frequent in pregnant women (Samorodinova et al. 1971; Nesbitt and Abdul-Karim 1982; Mlczoch et al. 1982). Mlczoch et al. (1982) present some data on the frequency and number of pregnancies in women over 16 years of age with congenital heart disease. Out of 261 women with congenital heart disease included in a 4-year prospective study, 147 had 303 pregnancies, 21 had no pregnancies in spite of a desire to have children, 64 had no wish to have children (either because of advanced age or because they were not married), and 29 women did not answer this question.

Contrary to the earlier opinion on the risk associated with pregnancy in women suffering from congenital heart disease, patients with acyanotic congenital heart disease quite often have uneventful pregnancies. This might be due to the adaptation of their cardiovascular system to various hemodynamic strains and overstrains in the very first years of their lives. In 1970 Neilson et al. reported their observations of 93 women with congenital (unoperated) heart disease who had 236 pregnancies, 3 maternal deaths, 23 miscarriages, and 213 deliveries of viable children. Other authors report similar data, except for Schaefer (1968), who out of 150 pregnancies in 51 women with congenital heart disease observed 20% of spontaneous abortions. He also examined a group of women who had undergone cardiac surgery before pregnancy. And though the defects had been successfully corrected, the prognosis for children of these women was worse than for children of healthy mothers. In the study performed by Mlczoch et al. (1982) fetal complications in 35 women operated for ventricular septal defect accounted for 34% and for 41% in 22 women with the same defect who were not operated upon, and vice versa 43% of maternal complications (dyspnea, edema, phlebitis, etc.) occurred in operated and 36% in unoperated women. In any case, it seems apparent that in many patients with congenital (and often also acquired) heart disease the fetus, to a certain extent, suffers from intrauterine hypoxia.

Such malformations as dextrocardia (without concomitant congenital heart disease, and anomaly of great arteries) and situs inversus completus do not usually have a detrimental effect on pregnancy, the latter in its turn having but a negligible effect on the cardiovascular system of such patients.

However, there are forms of congenital heart disease that put pregnant women at undoubted risk. These are primarily cyanotic forms of heart disease; primary pulmonary hypertension and severe pulmonary hypertension associated with Eisenmenger's syndrome; and severe coarctation of the aorta, aortic stenosis, and Marfan's syndrome with marked changes in the aortic root. The prognosis worsens in some pregnant women with patent ductus arteriousus and atrial and ventricular septal defects with reverse shunt if they have cyanosis and elevated pressure in the pulmonary circulation before pregnancy. Death in such patients during and after labor (sometimes also after termination of pregnancy) can be caused by severe cardiac or cardiopulmonary failure due to unfavorable blood redistribution between systemic and pulmonary circulation, abrupt shifts in the pressure gradient, and decompensated hypoxia. The prognosis can be worsened by the presence of systemic arterial hypertension, rupture of the aorta or arterial aneurysm, blood loss, and blood shunt reversion. The functional class is of high predictive value. In pulmonary hypertension the prognosis is, to a great extent, determined by the functional competence of the right ventricle. In severe pulmonary hypertension, systemic hypotension and cardiac output decrease in the intra- and postpartum periods can become life-threatening. In some forms of congenital heart disease acute cardiac failure develops immediately after delivery due to sudden decrease in the total peripheral vascular resistance paralleled by a decrease in pulmonary vascular resistance.

Subacute bacterial endocarditis, sometimes occurring in pregnant women with congenital heart disease, is associated with a serious risk. However, in spite of all the hazards favorable outcomes of pregnancy and delivery with uncomplicated postpartum period were reported even in women with Eisenmenger's syndrome, tetralogy of Fallot, Ebstein's anomaly, single ventricle, and primary pulmonary hypertension.

The patients with congenital heart disease develop compensatory shifts that should be considered in pregnancy. The anomalies associated with venous blood shunting into the arterial bed are accompanied by arterial hypoxemia, which above all can have an adverse effect on the fetus. However, compensatory mechanism triggered in these forms of the disease (polycythemia) increase blood volume and viscosity. An additional increase in BV during gestation threatens the onset of heart failure while increased blood viscosity is associated with a higher risk of thrombosis. A threat of pulmonary embolism is higher in heart failure, which is quite often accompanied by increased activity of the blood coagulation system, reduced activity of the anticoagulation system, and the formation of cardiac and vascular thrombi. Quite frequently patients with congenital heart disease develop cardiosclerosis, and pregnancy-induced myocardial overload in such cases can have a detrimental effect on circulation. Pulmonary hypertension in a number of congenital heart anomalies (including those with considerable left-to-right shunting) and in primary pulmonary vascular structural changes, poses a serious risk for pregnant women. At the same time, in the presence of mild to moderate left-to-right shunting, pregnancy-induced reduction in total peripheral resistance decreases blood shunting, while in cyanotic heart disease a reduced total peripheral resistance enhances right-to-left shunting and also cyanosis. Cyanotic forms of heart disease can be accompanied by a number of complications. But they do not arise in every patient and do not all necessarily occur in one patient. However, their likelihood should be taken into account and timely curative and preventive measures should be undertaken.

6.1.1 Atrial Septal Defect

Atrial septal defect is one of the commonest (9%–17%) defects observed in adult patients with congenital heart disease. It is $1\frac{1}{2}$–$3\frac{1}{2}$ times more frequent in females than in males and can have a familial character. A hemodynamically significant defect can be asymptomatic for many years. Starting with the 3rd or 4th decade physical exercise tolerance begins to diminish gradually. The incidence of complications also commences to rise during this period.

Depending on the location, atrial septal defects can be classified into ostium primum defects (20% of patients) and ostium secundum defects (80% of patients). Ostium primum defects are located in the lower part of the septum and can be associated with anomalous atrioventricular valves. Ostium secundum defects can be located in the posteroinferior, central, and posterosuperior septal areas and are frequently associated with anomalous pulmonary vein drainage into the right ventricle or vena cava. In uncomplicated defects left-to-right atrial shunting is present, which increases the right ventricular load and pulmonary blood flow. Pulmonary vasculature adapts to blood flow increase without pulmonary artery pressure elevation (only in the 5th decade does pulmonary vascular sclerosis begin to develop, pulmonary vascular resistance increase, and pulmonary hypertension develop; at this stage of the disease blood shunting is reversed). The right atrium, the pulmonary trunk, and its main branches are dilated.

The patients can remain asymptomatic for a long time; sometimes the patients complain of dyspnea on exertion and predisposition to respiratory infections. Inspection reveals pallor of the skin and sometimes cardiac "hump".

Palpation infrequently reveals intensified heart impulse, systolic impulse over the pulmonary artery area, and vibration due to pulmonic valve closure.

An auscultatory sign of the defect is a moderate systolic ejection murmur heard in the third and fourth left intercostal spaces (and the protodiastolic murmur peculiar to relative pulmonic valve incompetence). In rare cases the murmur is absent. The second heart sound over the pulmonary artery is split and intensified even in the absence of pulmonary hypertension. In ostium primum defect associated with mitral regurgitation holosystolic blowing murmur radiating into the axillary area is auscultated over the heart apex (in these cases intensified apex impulse and systolic thrill over the apex can be palpated). In the case of pulmonary hypertension (when marked cyanosis appears) the second heart sound accent over the pulmonary artery is increased; its splitting disappears and pulmonic valve opening click appears, soft protodiastolic blowing murmur of pulmonic valve insufficiency can be auscultated, and sometimes systolic murmur of tricuspid valve insufficiency is heard over the xiphoid process.

Peripheral pulse remains unchanged. Blood pressure and circulation time also remain practically unchanged. Venous pressure can be slightly elevated.

Cardiac size increases due to right heart chamber enlargement, intensified pulsation and dilatation of the main pulmonary artery, prominence of the main pulmonary artery, pulsation of hilar pulmonary arteries, and attenuated pulsation of the aorta; and increased pulmonary vascular markings are usually radiologically revealed. ECG exhibits rightward deviation of the electrical heart axis, often incomplete right bundle branch block, and sometimes first-degree atrioventricular block. In pulmonary hypertension high R_{V_1} and deep S_{V_6} waves appear. In patients over 30, atrial fibrillation or less frequently atrial flutter and paroxysmal supraventricular tachycardia can be recorded. Phonocardiogram registered in the second and third intercostal spaces reveals the second heart sound of increased intensity and systolic murmur.

Echocardiography reveals enlargement of the right ventricular cavity and paradoxical motion of the ventricular septum. Contrast echocardiography merely detects the shunting, while Doppler echocardiography enables one to assess its degree quantitatively. Heart catheterization and angiocardiographic findings are of great diagnostic value in unclear cases and when surgical intervention is considered.

The natural history of the disease can be complicated by pulmonary hypertension, right ventricular failure, thromboembolism (including paradoxical), and heart rhythm disturbances. Subacute bacterial endocarditis is an uncommon complication. The majority of patients with ostium secundum defect do accomodate well to hemodynamic overload associated with the first and repeated pregnancies. However, some authors (Mendelson 1960) report complicated and sometimes even fatal pregnancies in such patients: 11 of 88 pregnant women died, 9 of them of heart failure. The prognosis is certainly poorer in ostium primum defect (usually combined with mitral regurgitation) and in complicated forms of the defect: its combination with anomalous pulmonary vein drainage (10%–15% of cases), with mitral stenosis (Lutembacher's syndrome), or with marked heart rhythm disturbances.

During labor considerable blood loss can cause a fall in BP and reversed blood shunting leading to acute cyanosis. Reversed blood shunting can be also caused by postpartal pulmonary artery embolism, which can prove fatal.

6.1.2 Ventricular Septal Defect

Ventricular septal defect is one of the commonest (15%–29%) of the congenital heart anomalies, but less frequent in adults than atrial septal defect. It predominates in females. The defect can occupy the muscular, membranous (inferior to the crista supraventricularis), and subpulmonic (superior to the crista supraventricularis) region of the ventricular septum. In the latter case the defect is often associated with aortic valve incompetence. Membranous location of the defect is the most frequent.

The size, but not the location, of the defect is of hemodynamic importance. In mild to moderate defect (i.e., relatively small left-to-right shunting) pulmonary artery pressure either remains normal or is slightly elevated, irrespective of a considerable augmentation of the pulmonary blood flow. Further on, secondary pulmonary hypertension can develop. In large defect the prompt onset of secondary pulmonary hypertension is followed by heart failure (these patients do not usually reach childbearing age). Spontaneous closure of the defect is possible (usually a small defect in childhood).

The patients with small ventricular septal defects are usually asymptomatic and their inspection reveals no remarkable features. Large defects may be manifested in dyspnea and peripheral edema.

Palpation reveals intensified heart beat, and systolic thrill in the lower left parasternal area.

Auscultation detects accentuated and split second heart sound over the pulmonary artery and characteristic harsh holosystolic murmur audible in the majority of cases in the third and fourth left intercostal spaces (or in the first and second intercostal spaces — in subpulmonic defect). In large defects the murmur is very harsh and widespread. As pulmonary hypertension progresses, the murmur intensity can reduce and blowing diastolic murmur over the pulmonic valve becomes audible (at this stage the shunt becomes bidirectional, which is the reason for the appearance of cyanosis).

Peripheral pulse, arterial and venous pressure, and circulation time remain practically unchanged.

Roentgenological findings in patients with small ventricular septal defects reveal practically no changes of the heart shadow. In large shunts the increase first in the left ventricular and left atrial and then in right ventricular size, as well as prominence of the main pulmonary segment, pronounced pulsation of the hilar pulmonary arteries, and increased pulmonary arterial vasculature are noted.

Electrocardiography in patients with small defects is normal. Increased left-to-right shunting can give rise to left ventricular hypertrophy signs and the onset of pulmonary hypertension to right ventricular hypertrophy signs. Arrhythmias and conduction disturbances are not characteristic of ventricular septal defect.

Phonocardiographic and auscultatory findings are identical. When the recordings are performed in the third or fourth intercostal spaces, loud holosystolic murmur can engulf both the first and second heart sounds.

In moderate to large ventricular septal defect two-dimensional echocardiography records the echo signal absence in the affected area, and left and right ventricular as well as left atrial enlargement. Contrast echocardiography reveals the presence of blood shunting, while Doppler echocardiography permits quantitative assessment of its degree.

Heart catheterization and angiocardiography determine the volume of blood shunting and the magnitude of the defect; after that the indications for surgical interventions may be considered.

The disease can be complicated by severe pulmonary hypertension, right ventricular failure, and subacute bacterial endocarditis. Women with small ventricular septal defects usually tolerate pregnancy well. In large ventricular septal defect pregnancy-induced BV increase can cause heart failure, sometimes fatal. Paradoxical systemic embolism through ventricular septal defect may develop in the early puerperium. In the early puerperium, as in the case of atrial septal defect, there is a risk of blood shunting reversion accompanied by acute cyanosis in cases of a dramatic BP fall caused by considerable blood loss.

6.1.3 Patent Ductus Arteriosus

Ductus arteriosus is a normal embryonic vessel connecting the descending aorta with the pulmonary artery. It is usually obliterated shortly after birth and failure of ductus closure is an anomaly causing blood shunting from the aorta into the pulmonary artery. A small patent ductus arteriosus causes no changes of the heart. However, in large left-to-right shunting pulmonary artery, left ventricle and left atrium are dilated. With increased pulmonary vascular resistance, pulmonary hypertension and right ventricular overload develop. Right-to-left shunting is infrequent. The defect occurs with a frequency two to three times higher in females than in males. In recent years the incidence of patent ductus arteriosus in pregnant women has become lower, since surgical closure of the defect is mostly performed in childhood.

The patients with small patent ductus arteriosus produce no symptoms. In considerable blood shunting they experience fatigability and dyspnea on exertion. Inspection of the patients reveals no specific features.

Palpation in the second left intercostal space usually reveals systolic or continuous thrill.

Characteristic continuous murmur of patent ductus arteriosus, the harsh so-called "machinery" or "clattering" murmur, is maximal in the second (sometimes first) left intercostal space. In small ductus arteriosus only systolic murmur is audible. The murmur is attenuated in pulmonary hypertension development and is intensified in response to pressor amine administration.

The peripheral arterial pulse can be bounding (prompt rise and fall). Systolic BP is somewhat elevated or normal, while there is a significant fall in diastolic pressure. Venous pressure remains virtually unchanged.

Heart size on radiological examination may be within normal limits, but more often left atrial or left ventricular enlargement is observed. The pulmonary artery segment of the left heart border is prominent. Unlike ventricular and artrial septal defects, the aortic arch is also prominent. Pulsation of both vessels is increased.

The electrocardiogram records the signs of left ventricular overload in the presence of a large left-to-right shunting or signs of right or left and right ventricular overload in the presence of pulmonary hypertension.

The phonocardiogram recorded in the second left intercostal space reveals an increased amplitude of the second heart sound, and continuous murmur with the maximal amplitude in mid or late systole (the amplitude is minimal in late diastole or early systole).

Heart catheterization and angiocardiography are performed only in diagnostically obscure cases and when surgical treatment is considered.

The disease can be complicated by pulmonary hypertension and reversed shunting, acute bacterial endocarditis, and heart failure.

In small or moderate blood shunting pregnancy does not aggravate the course of the disease. Maternal mortality in uncomplicated patent ductus arteriosus does not exceed 0.6% (Jones and Howitt 1965). Large blood shunting is a threat of left ventricular failure caused partly by pregnancy-induced BV increase. At the early stages of pulmonary hypertension a rise in pulmonary artery pressure can lead to right ventricular failure during pregnancy. As in cases of atrial and ventricular septal defects, substantial blood loss with associated BP fall may result in blood shunting reversion. In rare cases pulmonary artery embolism and the rupture of pulmonary artery aneurysm can occur during gestation (Szekeli and Snaith 1974).

6.1.4 Valvular Pulmonic Stenosis

Isolated valvular pulmonic stenosis comprises 8%–10% of the total number of cases of congenital heart disease. The narrowing is commonly due to valve cusp commissural fusion forming a dome-shaped diaphragm with a small orifice. It is more seldom that the infundibular stenosis is caused by fibromuscular collar in the distal part of the right ventricular outflow tract. The root of the pulmonary trunk is characterized by poststenotic dilatation. Valvular pulmonic stenosis is infrequently associated with ventricular septal defect.

The hemodynamic consequence of right ventricular outflow tract narrowing is the pressure gradient between the ventricle and the pulmonary artery. Systolic pressure elevation leads to right ventricular hypertrophy with following dilatation; right atrial pressure increases. This may be followed by the opening of the foramen ovale in the atrial septum and right-to-left blood shunting.

The patients complain of fatigue, dyspnea (initially on exertion and ultimately at rest), dizziness, and sometimes syncope. Inspection of patients reveals cyanosis in the presence of patent foramen ovale. Sometimes cardiac "hump" is observed.

Palpation reveals an increased heart impulse and sometimes systolic thrill in the second and third left intercostal spaces.

Auscultation reveals attenuated second heart sound over the pulmonary artery and characteristic harsh systolic murmur in the second and third left intercostal spaces (or in the third and fourth left intercostal spaces in infundibular stenosis) with radiation into the left intraclavicular area. In mild to moderate stenosis the murmur is soft and systolic click is audible.

Peripheral pulse and blood pressure remain practically unchanged. Venous pressure in severe cases is elevated.

The chest roentgenogram in mild stenosis reveals normal or slightly increased heart size and shows some prominence of the main pulmonary artery (except cases of infundibular stenosis), indicating poststenotic dilatation. In marked stenosis the right ventricle is often enlarged and in severe obstruction right atrial prominence is observed. The pulmonary vascular pattern is usually decreased.

The electrocardiogram exhibits rightward deviation of the electrical heart axis and, in severe cases, signs of right ventricular hypertrophy and sometimes right atrial overload.

The phonocardiogram records split and attenuated second heart sound over the pulmonary artery and systolic murmur whose duration in moderate stenosis is limited by the aortic component of the second heart sound, while in severe cases the murmur is of longer duration.

Heart catheterization and angiocardiography are performed when surgical correction is being considered.

The disease may be complicated by right ventricular failure (caused in pregnancy by BV and cardiac output increase) and subacute bacterial endocarditis. Valvalur pulmonic stenosis is characterized by a rather high incidence of premature labor (Mlczoch et al. 1982).

6.1.5 Tetralogy of Fallot

Tetralogy of Fallot is a classic cyanotic congenital heart disease comprising about 7%–8% of all congenital heart malformations encountered in adults. The defect is caused by pulmonic stenosis (more often subvalvular), large ventricular septal defect, dextroposition of the aorta, and right ventricular hypertrophy.

Hemodynamic shifts are induced by ventricular septal defect and pulmonic stenosis. In a very large defect right and left ventricular pressures can equalize. Blood shunting direction is dependent on the degree of right ventricular outflow tract obstruction; in severe cases the venous blood flows into the aorta; in mild stenosis there is left-to-right shunting (as in ordinary ventricular septal defect). In the latter case acyanotic or "pink" form of tetralogy of Fallot is observed. In right ventricular outflow obstruction pregnancy-induced drop in peripheral vascular resistance and an increase in cardiac output and venous return result in larger right-to-left shunting, a fall in systemic arterial oxygen saturation, deeper cyanosis, and also a rise in hematocrit.

Clinical manifestations of acyanotic tetralogy of Fallot are similar to those of ventricular septal defect or pulmonary artery stenosis. The patients with cyanotic forms of the defect complain of fatigability even on mild exertion, dizziness, dyspnea on exertion, and sometimes syncope. On inspection, cyanotic mucous membranes and skin, clubbing of the fingers, retarded growth, and sometimes cardiac "hump" are apparent.

Physical findings on palpation include intensified heart impulse and occasionally systolic thrill in the second and third left intercostal spaces.

Harsh systolic murmur is audible in the third and fourth left intercostal spaces. Its intensity inversely correlates with the magnitude of ventricular septal defect. The murmur increases after phenylephrine injection and attenuates after amylnitrite inhalation.

No significant changes in heart size are visible on posteroanterior chest films; sometimes the so-called coeur en sabot contour is noted: moderate leftward deviation of a somewhat sharpened and uplifted left ventricular contour with concave main pulmonary artery segment. In the right anterior oblique projection right ventricular enlargement is observed. In severe pulmonic stenosis the aortic arch is prominent.

Pulmonary vasculature usually decreases; however, with well-developed bronchial collaterals it may increase.

The electrocardiogram demonstrates the pattern of right ventricular hypertrophy. The pattern of left ventricular hypertrophy can be revealed in well-developed collateral circulation and increased pulmonary blood flow.

The phonocardiogram records second heart sound splitting and attenuation of its pulmonary component; systolic murmur in the third and fourth left intercostal spaces is maximal in early systole.

Echocardiography demonstrates the disappearance of echo signals from the area of ventricular septal defect, anomalous forward displacement of the aorta, right ventricular enlargement, ventricular septum thickening, and dilatation of the aorta.

Clinical blood examinations show the presence of polycythemia.

Heart catheterization and angiocardiography are most informative for the diagnosis of tetralogy of Fallot.

The complications of tetralogy of Fallot are as follows: cerebral hypoxia and cerebral thrombosis, subacute bacterial endocarditis, and heart failure. In pregnancy the risk of complications is considerably increased. Pregnancy in women with tetralogy of Fallot imposes a significant threat for the mother and fetus. Prognosis is unfavorable in repeated syncope, a rise in hematocrit over 60%, peripheral arterial oxygen saturation below 80%, and right ventricular pressure above 120 mmHg (Jacoby 1964). Abrupt hemodynamic fluctuations during labor pose a serious risk for patients with tetralogy of Fallot. In the early puerperium there is the greatest risk of severe syncope. Due to high right ventricular pressure sudden abrupt drop in systemic and left ventricular pressure immediately after labor is associated with a greater threat than in patients with left-to-right blood shunting. Mendelson (1960) in his summarized data obtained in a number of investigations of pregnant women with tetralogy of Fallot reported the development of heart failure in 40%, maternal mortality in 12%, and fetal loss in 36% of cases. Pregnant women with tetralogy of Fallot have a high incidence of spontaneous abortions, stillbirths, premature labor, and at term delivery of children with low birth weight. However, exceptional cases do occur; Shrestna et al. (1979) have reported a patient with tetralogy of Fallot who has safely given birth to five children.

6.1.6 Eisenmenger's Syndrome

Eisenmenger's syndrome is included in the cyanotic congenital heart malformations though it cannot be considered an individual nosological form. Eisenmenger's syndrome is an association of a congenital communication between the systemic and pulmonary circuits with severe pulmonary hypertension due to high pulmonary vascular resistance. It occurs in large septal defects and large communication between the aorta and the pulmonary artery (i.e., in ventricular and atrial septal defects and patent ductus arteriosus). In all the cases there are considerable changes in the pulmonary vessel walls.

As the syndrome progresses, the increase in pulmonary vascular resistance leads to a reduction in left-to-right shunting and pulmonary artery pressure elevation. With pulmonary artery pressure equal or even greater than systemic pressure, the shunt becomes bidirectional or reverses completely to right-to-left.

In left-to-right blood shunting the patients can remain asymptomatic for a long period. Later they may experience fatigability and dyspnea. The incidence and increase of cyanosis, polycythemia, and clubbing tend to increase with age. Syncope, hemoptysis, and chest pain are observed.

Clinical findings of right ventricular hypertrophy, loud second heart sound at the pulmonary area, and widespread systolic murmur along the left sternal edge are common. In some cases blowing diastolic murmur of pulmonary regurgitation or systolic murmur of tricuspid regurgitation can be heard. Pulmonary artery valve opening snap and the third and fourth heart sounds may be revealed. Venous pressure is usually normal.

Roentgenological findings of the heart size are often normal (marked cardiomegaly is present in atrial septal defect); however, right ventricular hypertrophy or dilatation can be revealed. Prominence of the aortic knob suggests patent ductus arteriosus. Calcification of the ductus arteriosus or pulmonary artery may be visible. Dilatation of the main pulmonary artery and its proximal branches with diminished vascular markings in the peripheral lung fields may be seen.

The electrocardiogram demonstrates signs of right atrial overload and right ventricular hypertrophy. In some cases in the presence of ventricular septal defects or patent ductus arteriosus signs of left ventricular hypertrophy are seen.

Heart catheterization and angiocardiography are essential for the detection of the defects.

Eisenmenger's syndrome is often complicated by: thrombosis in the pulmonary artery system, cerebral thrombosis, subacute bacterial endocarditis, and heart failure. Sudden death may occur. Pregnancy in women with Eisenmenger's syndrome is associated with increased risk; the higher the pulmonary artery pressure, the greater the risk. Hemoptysis may first appear during gestation. Pregnancy is not associated with a parallel reduction in total and pulmonary vascular resistance, resulting in larger right-to-left shunting, reduced pulmonary blood flow, a drop in arterial oxygen saturation, and a rise in hematocrit. If hematocrit exceeds 60%, the fetus dies (Arnon and Steinfeld 1985). A sudden rise in pulmonary vascular resistance or a decrease in total peripheral resistance leading to preload reduction during labor or immediately after delivery impose still greater threats. In both cases a severe collapse can ensue as a result of abrupt BP fall. Expulsive efforts can be accompanied by the increase in the peripheral vascular resistance leading to cardiac output decrease that also gives rise to severe collapse. Preeclampsia-eclampsia can aggravate the hemodynamic situation due to abrupt shifts in peripheral vascular resistance. Moreover, considerable physical exertion in Eisenmenger's syndrome can induce a dramatic rise in right ventricular pressure that may provoke fatal arrhythmias. There is also a persistent risk of severe syncope and pulmonary thromboembolism. Maternal mortality in Eisenmenger's syndrome is estimated as very high (Maarek-Charbit and Corone 1986). Fetal loss in mothers with Eisenmenger's syndrome is also very high. Batson (1974) reports a 33% fetal loss in 10 sick women with 23 pregnancies, but no maternal deaths have been registered in this study. Women with this syndrome seldom have full-term pregnancies. The incidence of spontaneous abortions approaches 43% (Mlczoch et al. 1982). Most findings observed in Eisenmenger's syndrome hold true for primary pulmonary hypertension.

6.1.7 Congenital Aortic Stenosis

Congenital obstruction of the left ventricular outflow tract can be subvalvular, valvular, and supravalvular. Congenital forms of aortic stenosis are observed in 3%–11% of patients with congenital heart defects. Congenital valvular and subvalvular aortic stenosis have much in common, although there are certain features peculiar to supravalvular stenosis. In the majority of cases congenital stenosis is valvular. Though this form of the disease is usually fairly well tolerated by adults, there is a gradual increase in the degree of outflow obstruction in most cases.

The commissures of the abnormal valve are fused. The valve is thickened and dome-shaped with a small orifice. In severe stenosis, concentric left ventricular hypertrophy without considerable changes in the size of the ventricular cavity is present, and ascending aorta becomes poststenotically dilated. In subvalvular stenosis outflow tract narrowing is caused either by a discrete fibrous collar located immediately under the valve cusps or by a thick fibromuscular ring located at a slightly lower level. Both forms of stenosis can be coupled with coarctation of the aorta or patent ductus arteriosus. In supravalvular aortic stenosis the obstruction is distal to Valsalva sinuses. The hourglass type of deformity is the most common. In other cases either diaphragm-like stenosis or diffuse narrowing of the ascending aorta may be observed. Poststenotic dilatation of the aorta is never observed in supravalvular stenosis; however, its wall can be thickened.

A hemodynamic manifestation of the defect is a systolic pressure gradient between the left ventricle and the aorta (between the aortic root and ascending aorta in supravalvular stenosis), which depends on stroke volume, ejection time, and degree of obstruction. In advanced stages characterized by heart failure, left ventricular dilatation develops; left ventricular, left atrial, and pulmonary venous end-diastolic pressures rise (possibly causing pulmonary edema); and in severe cases pulmonary hypertension and right ventricular failure can ensue.

Pregnancy-induced BV and stroke volume increase contribute to the rise in transaortic pressure gradient, systolic left ventricular pressure, and left ventricular work and can occasionally give rise to heart failure.

Clinical and laboratory findings of congenital valvular aortic stenosis are identical to those of rheumatic aortic stenosis. History data and signs of associated heart diseases (in acquired heart disease rheumatic lesions of other, usually mitral, heart valves are frequent; in congenital aortic stenosis other congenital cardiovascular lesions are seldom observed) are essential for the differential diagnosis of the disease.

In subvalvular stenosis systolic murmur in some cases can be better auscultated not in the right but in the left third and fourth intercostal spaces. The ejection click often audible in mild or moderate valvular stenosis is absent in the subvalvular form; poststenotic dilatation of the aorta and calcification of the aortic valve cusps are never observed. The chest roentgenogram more often demonstrates normal heart size in patients with congenital than with acquired stenosis if heart failure is not present.

Supravalvular aortic stenosis may be familial; the hypercalcemia syndrome is either observed in history or detected during examination. In the predominant diaphragmal form of stenosis the patients have a typical appearance (overhanging upper lip, low positioned ears, epicanthal folds, strabismus, dental hypoplasia) and mental retardation. Unlike valvular stenosis, in supravalvular stenosis the second heart sound can be intensified, and in addition systolic thrill and systolic murmur in some cases are clearly revealed only along the right sternal edge (systolic murmur is well transmitted also to the carotid arteries). The pressure difference in the contralateral brachial and radial arteries is typical (pulsation is more prominent and the pressure is higher on the right than on the left side). About 30% of patients with supravalvular aortic stenosis show stenotic pulmonary artery branches.

Quite often it is possible to identify the site of obstruction to the left ventricular outflow only by heart catheterization and angiocardiography. It is essential to differentiate congenital valvular aortic stenosis from rheumatic aortic stenosis and idiopathic hypertrophic subaortic stenosis, as management of these conditions is different.

Pregnant women with mild to moderate congenital aortic stenosis tolerate pregnancy fairly well; however, the risk of subacute bacterial endocarditis in the puerperium is independent of the degree of stenosis. Sometimes syncope caused by aortic stenosis and occurring with physical exertion and nervous excitement may first appear in gestation. Cerebral symptoms, dyspnea, and retrosternal pain in early pregnancy expose the patients to the risk of serious complications (Perloff 1984) including acute heart failure and sudden death (caused mainly by asystolia and ventricular fibrillation).

6.1.8 Coarctation of the Aorta (Aortic Isthmus Stenosis)

Though congenital narrowing may occur at any portion along the aorta, the defect in 95% of cases is located in the isthmus as a rule distal to the left subclavian artery. Occasionally, there is no opening at all. The aortic dilatation is usually poststenotic, although prestenotic dilatation is also possible. The development of collaterals along normal intervascular arterial anastomoses arising from the aorta proximally and distally to coarctation is characteristic of the defect (internal mammary, intercostal and scapular arteries are essential). In adults degenerative changes (friability, fibrosis, calcification) may be present in aortic regions proximal and distal to coarctation, which are commonly accompanied by the formation of aneurysm (in collateral vessels as well). There is an opinion that pregnancy causes changes in the media of the aorta, contributing to its dissection and even rupture. The aneurysms of the circle of Willis are considered a risk factor in some patients with coarctation of the aorta.

Hemodynamic sequelae of blood flow obstruction in the aorta are systolic left ventricular pressure elevation and marked blood pressure increase in all the arterial branches proximal to coarctation (kidney ischemia also plays a certain role in the development of hypertension). Blood pressure in the arteries distal to coarctation is normal, somewhat reduced (only systolic pressure) or elevated. Coarctation of the aorta is frequently associated with a bicuspid aortic valve.

Coarctation of the aorta is encountered in almost 10% of pregnant women with congenital heart and great vessel malformations (Nesbitt and Abdul-Karim 1982). Pregnancy-induced BV and cardiac output increase does not always entail a rise in the already elevated BP, as there is a parallel drop in peripheral vascular resistance in gestation. An additional BP elevation occurs somewhat more often by the end of the gestational period or during labor.

The patients with coarctation of the aorta are commonly asymptomatic. Sometimes they complain of headache, nasal hemorrhages, mild dyspnea, fatigue or pain in the legs upon physical exertion, and foot sensitivity to cold. On inspection pulsation of the aortic arch can be seen in some patients in the retrosternal notch. With the development of collaterals, their pulsation can become visible in the scapular or posterior intercostal regions, especially with the patient in a sitting-stooping position.

On palpation there is an intensified (not always) apical impulse in its usual place. Pulsation of the intercostal and scapular arteries is often revealed. In the left second intercostal space, systolic murmur transmitted to neck vessels and interscapular region is auscultated. An aortic systolic ejection click is in some cases heard at the heart apex. The murmur can be audible also over intercostal and scapular arteries.

Pulsation of the radial arteries is strong, while in the femoral arteries it is either weak or altogether absent. The femoral pulse, if any, is delayed in comparison with the brachial artery pulse. Marked systolic blood pressure elevation in the arms with blood pressure in the legs either reduced or the same (normally, BP in the lower extremities is higher than in the upper extremities by 10–20 mm Hg) is believed to be a specific feature of coarctation of the aorta. Diastolic pressure is normal or moderately elevated. As a result, pulse pressure is high in the arms and low in the legs. Sometimes resting BP in the arms is normal, but it rises abruptly in response to physical exertion. If the left subclavian artery originates from the aorta at the site of the obstruction or distally to it, the left radial artery pulse will be attenuated (or even absent) and BP will be lower in the left rather than in the right arm. Venous pressure remains normal.

On chest radiograms heart size and contours are often normal, or sometimes enlarged due to left ventricular hypertrophy. Notching of the inferior margins of posterior rib segments due to the compression by the arterial collaterals is a common radiographic feature. The barium esophagogram may reveal displacement of the esophagus by a dilated aorta above and below the site of coarctation. The degree and location of the aortic narrowing are specified by aortography.

The electrocardiogram is normal or reflects some degree of left ventricular hypertrophy. The phonocardiogram records accentuated second heart sound over the aorta and widespread systolic murmur originating in midsystole. The bicuspid aortic valve can be detected echocardiographically.

Heart catheterization and angiocardiography are performed in suspected coexisting heart malformations.

Coarctation of the aorta can be complicated by left ventricular failure with pulmonary edema, hypertensive encephalopathy, stroke (often caused by aneurysm rupture in the arteris of the circle of Willis), subacute bacterial endocarditis (especially in coarctation of the aorta coupled with the bicuspid aortic valve), dissection, or rupture of the aorta. All these complications can occur in pregnant women, whose mortality rate in this defect is 3.5%–9% (a higher mortality rate is caused by combined heart disease). The most common cause of death, according to Goodwin (1961), is rupture of the aorta (usually proximal to coarctation). Complications occur more frequently in the third trimester of pregnancy and immediately near term, although they can also occur during labor.

6.1.9 Uncommon Congenital Heart Defects

6.1.9.1 Ebstein's Anomaly

Ebstein's anomaly is caused by displacement of one or two tricuspid valve leaflets into the right ventricle often accompanied by their degenerative changes. As a result, tricuspid insufficiency and atrialization with thinning of the supravalvular part of the right ventricle take place. This anomaly can be coupled with atrial septal defect. In large atrial septal defect right-to-left shunting may develop.

The anomaly is sometimes manifested in dyspnea, palpitation, and cyanosis. The third and fourth heart sounds, systolic murmur of tricuspid insufficiency, and sometimes diastolic murmur of relative tricuspid stenosis are audible. Paroxysms of supraventricular tachycardia and episodes of atrial flutter and fibrillation are frequent. Clinical symptoms of the Wolff-Parkinson-White syndrome can first appear in pregnancy.

The electrocardiogram exhibits a prolonged P-Q interval and signs of right ventricular overload, and right bundle branch block. Echocardiography reveals right ventricular enlargement and delayed tricuspid valve closure in comparison with mitral valve closure. Blood shunting can be determined by contrast and Doppler echocardiography.

Though there are reports of successful delivery in women with Ebstein's anomaly, the presence of this disease in pregnant women is associated with considerable risk. The small, functionally incompetent, and already overloaded right ventricle copes poorly with pregnancy-induced increase in BV. This may result in right ventricular failure. Attacks of arrhythmia are poorly tolerated in pregnancy. In the presence of atrial septal defect cyanosis caused by reversed blood shunting can first appear during pregnancy due to the reduction in the peripheral vascular resistance, tachycardia, and right ventricular overload. Pregnancy in these cases increases the risk of parodoxical cerebral embolism through the defect. The incidence of spontaneous abortions is high in cyanotic patients with Ebstein's anomaly.

6.1.9.2 Congenital Complete Heart Block

Familial congenital heart block is diagnosed if there are documented history data of the time of its onset. It is usually isolated, although it can be coupled with other cardiovascular anomalies (corrected transposition of great vessels or ventricular septal defect). Unlike patients with acquired complete heart block, the patients with congenital isolated block have a higher heart rate (50 beats/min), less frequently experience Adams-Stokes attacks, and can lead a normal active life. In some patients the ventricular rate can increase with exertion and after atropine injection.

The patients are usually asymptomatic. The electrocardiogram in the majority of cases records normal QRS complexes supraventricular in origin (the prognosis is complicated when QRS complexes are broadened and the ventricular rate is slow).

Pregnancy and labor in congenital complete heart block are usually uneventful (the heart augments the stroke volume), though in some women Adams-Stokes attacks may first appear during pregnancy and labor. On rare occasions heart failure develops. Fetal loss in women with congenital complete heart block is rather high.

6.1.9.3 Bicuspid Aortic Valve

Bicuspid aortic valve is rarely diagnosed as this anomaly has no hemodynamic or clinical manifestations. Roberts (1970) regards it as one of the commonest congenital valvular anomalies. The aortic valve has only two cusps of unequal sizes with one commissure. A rudimentary third cusp may be present. The prolapse of the larger cusp into the aorta during systole may be the cause of congenital aortic incompetence having the same clinical features as the acquired regurgitation. Valvular regurgitation may also develop if there is a small ventricular septal defect at the site of the cusp attachement leading to cusp prolapse. The cusps may become fibrous, thickened, and calcified over the years, which gives rise to valvular aortic stenosis with a typical clinical picture. However, in some cases systolic murmur in the second right intercostal space without any other clinical and hemodynamic shifts typical of aortic stenosis can appear in unchanged cusps. Bicuspid aortic valve is often coupled with coarctation of the aorta and patent ductus arteriosus. And, finally, what is essential for pregnant women, it often becomes a site of subacute bacterial endocarditis. The isolated anomaly with normal valve function often remains undetected in young women prior to or during pregnancy; however, the appearance of valvular regurgitation in the puerperium can be the consequence of bacterial endocarditis.

In mild to moderate congenital aortic regurgitation pregnancy is usually tolerated fairly well, as heart work increase due to cardiac output elevation is to a certain extent compensated by peripheral vascular resistance reduction, and because heart rate increase shortens diastole and leads to the decrease of regurgitation. However, if a woman had marked clinical manifestations of aortic regurgitation (including end-diastolic left ventricular pressure elevation) severe left ventricular failure may develop in gestation. Patients with bicuspid aortic valve are predisposed to aortic dissection. Bicuspid aortic valve can be diagnosed by means of echocardiography, biplane angiography of the aortic root, and left ventriculography.

6.1.9.4 Primary Pulmonary Hypertension

Primary pulmonary hypertension is an uncommon disease of unknown etiology, its incidence being five times higher in females than in males.

The patients usually complain of dyspnea on exertion (eventually also at rest), weakness, chest pain (sometimes irradiating to the neck), palpitation, syncope, cough, and hemoptysis. On inspection (and/or on palpation) intensified right ventricular pulsation can be revealed to the left of the sternum, and pulsation of the dilated pulmonary artery in the second left intercostal space is detected. Systolic murmur and sometimes a systolic click is also heard in the second left intercostal space. The second heart sound is split especially at the pulmonary artery area. The fourth heart sound is audible at times. At advanced stages there are features of right ventricular failure. In severe pulmonary hypertension the third heart sound, holosystolic murmur, and early diastolic murmur at the pulmonary artery area are heard.

The electrocardiogram shows the pattern of right atrial and ventricular hypertrophy. Radiographically, dilation of the main pulmonary artery and its both great branches as well as the enlargement of the right atrium and ventricle are revealed. Echocardiography in addition to right heart hypertrophy demonstrates ventricular septal thickening.

Hemodynamic shifts peculiar to pregnancy have an adverse effect on patients with primary pulmonary hypertension. Cardiac output increase leading to venous return elevation augments the load on the right ventricle that works against high pulmonary vascular resistance, which unlike systemic vascular resistance is not reduced in pregnancy. Augmented blood volume aggravates the situation.

Sometimes pregnancy worsens the condition of patients with pulmonary hypertension who in the prepregnancy period revealed no clinical manifestations of the disease. Gestation frequently worsens the already existing symptoms of the disease (dyspnea, syncope, chest pain, etc.). Labor and the puerperium are associated with greater risk than pregnancy per se. Sudden death may occur. Maternal mortality can reach 50% (Szekely and Snaith 1974).

6.2 Mitral Valve Prolapse

Mitral valve prolapse may be congenital (primary and in the Ehlers-Danlos and Marfan's syndromes) and acquired (in rheumatic endocarditis, hypertrophic subaortic stenosis, congestive cardiomyopathy, myocarditis, some congenital heart diseases, systemic lupus erythematosus, periarteritis nodosa and other diseases, or following blunt heart trauma and mitral valve surgery). In recent years, with the use of echocardiography (if its criteria are correct), it became possible to identify this syndrome in 5%–10% of the total population examined, with it predominating in females. The disease can be hereditary. Mitral valvular apparatus defect is manifested in the prolapse of one (or sometimes both) of the leaflets during systole into the left atrium, giving rise to blood regurgitation into the atrium. The primary syndrome is characterized by myxomatous changes of the mitral complex due to collagen metabolism disturbances; other heart valves (aortic and tricuspid) may also be involved. It is thought that posterior leaflet prolapse can provoke reflectory spasm of normal coronary arteries, with arising myocardial ischemia probably being the cause of angina pectoris, myocardial infarction, arrhythmias, and sudden death (Braunwald 1984).

Hemodynamic shifts are caused by mitral regurgitation. The preload increase in pregnancy has a favorable effect, while inotropism elevation and afterload reduction are unfavorable (Sullivan and Ramanathan 1985).

There may be cases of sudden death of the patients' relatives in the history. The majority of patients with mitral valve prolapse are asymptomatic. In some cases they complain of anxiety, palpitation, and unpleasant sensation in the chest (from feelings of discomfort to typical anginal pain not always associated with exertion, and acute stabbing pain attacks at the heart apex area).

Inspection and palpation are unremarkable in the absence of associated heart diseases and marked regurgitation, but the patients are frequently asthenic. A characteristic feature of mitral valve prolapse is a midsystolic click, in the majority of cases accompanied by late systolic murmur clearly audible in the fourth and fifth left intercostal spaces. In severe regurgitation the murmur is holosystolic. Some patients reveal only one of these auscultatory findings that may sometimes temporarily disappear. In Valsalva maneuver the murmur is not intensified, but becomes more durable; squatting shortens and attenuates the murmur and standing up prolongs and intensifies the murmur. Leaflet prolapse is well detected by angiocardiography.

The electrocardiogram of asymptomatic patients having auscultatory signs of mitral valve prolapse can be normal. More often nonspecific ST segment changes and inverted or diphasic T waves are recorded in leads II, III, and aVF. These changes become more pronounced (or sometimes first appear) during physical exercise or amylnitrite inhalation. Arrhythmias (atrial and ventricular premature beats, supraventricular and ventricular tachycardia, bradyarrhythmia, and AV block of varying degree) are often detected. Refractory ventricular tachycardia that can be transformed into ventricular fibrillation constitutes a major threat.

The phonocardiogram findings usually correspond to the auscultatory data. The click of mitral valve prolapse differs from the ejection click in that it appears 0.14 s after the first heart sound (after the carotid pulse begins to rise). Systolic murmur begins in mid- or late systole and is of increasing intensity.

The echocardiogram registers an abrupt backward motion of the posterior mitral valve leaflet (both leaflets) in early and midsystole, systolic prolapse of posterior (or both) leaflets, or occasionally rapid backward motion of the anterior leaflet. In some cases, in spite of systolic click and murmur, the echocardiogram may be normal and vice versa. Echocardiographic findings of mitral valve prolapse are present in almost all the patients with Marfan's syndrome. Myxomatous changes of the mitral valve are echocardiographically revealed in these patients.

The following complications can be observed: increasing valvular regurgitation, paroxysmal arrhythmias, transitory acute hemiplegia (resulting from microembolism), cerebral infarction (seldom), and subacute bacterial endocarditis.

In patients with Marfan's syndrome myxomatous mitral and aortic valve degeneration is associated with thinned and prolonged valvular chordae tendineae; the mitral valve ring, aortic sinuses, and aortic root are dilated.

Increased cardiac output and reduced peripheral vascular resistance in pregnancy can decrease the degree of mitral valve prolapse. In such cases, the systolic click and late systolic murmur are weak or disappear altogether and in the absence of characteristic echocardiographic findings, mitral valve prolapse is impossible to diagnose. After delivery auscultatory phenomena reappear. Pregnancy increases the risk of subacute endocarditis and rupture of valvular chordae tendineae (especially during labor). Paroxysms of arrhythmias (namely supraventricular tachycardia), most undesirable during labor, become more frequent in gestation. However, some authors (Rayburn and Fontana 1981; Shapiro et al. 1985; Plotti et al. 1985) report pregnant women with mitral valve prolapse who had uncomplicated full-term pregnancies and labor of normal duration and gave birth to offsprings of normal weight. With pronounced mitral valve prolapse dyspnea may be increased and arrhythmias may become more frequent. Prospective echocardiographic study has revealed an increase in the degree of mitral valve prolapse in the postpartal period (Titchenko 1985).

7 Diseases of the Myocardium, Endocardium, and Pericardium and Uncommon Heart Diseases in Pregnancy

7.1 Diseases of the Myocardium

7.1.1 Myocarditis

Myocarditis of different etiology is at present rather seldom observed in pregnancy. Up to the 1960s–1970s recurrence of rheumatic carditis predominated. In the past decade due to a milder course of rheumatic fever and efficient preventive treatment of rheumatic patients, postinfective (caused by respiratory infections) myocarditis, which sometimes remains undiagnosed because of its mild course, has been relatively more frequent. It is difficult to predict the course of myocarditis in pregnancy: in some cases heart failure or embolism can develop, or severe acute myocarditis may sometimes be the cause of sudden death (Burch 1977). This does not mean that termination of pregnancy is necessarily indicated in patients with myocarditis. The prognosis and management depend on the etiology, severity, and stage of myocarditis, its previous recurrence, and the possible presence of valvular heart disease. It should be remembered that rheumatic carditis can recur in the postpartum period and can prove fatal (Szekely and Snaith 1974).

7.1.1.1 Rheumatic Carditis

Certain immunity disturbances during gestation (especially in complicated pregnancy) can lead to the exacerbation of the rheumatic process even after a slight cold or the recurrence of chronic tonsillitis. Myocarditis in rheumatic fever exacerbation is commonly coupled with endocarditis.

Clinical symptoms and signs of rheumatic carditis in pregnancy are the same as in nonpregnant patients. Such complaints as precordial discomfort, dyspnea on exertion, as well as subfebrile temperature are not pathognomonic because they can be induced by pregnancy. Articular manifestations of the disease are seldom observed.

Primary rheumatic carditis is nowadays infrequent in pregnancy, and, therefore, in exacerbations of rheumatic carditis manifestations of an existing rheumatic valvular disease are revealed on examination. In primary rheumatic carditis heart sounds are somewhat muffled; the third and fourth heart sounds may appear. A faint systolic murmur is commonly heard over the heart apex (in pronounced endocardial lesions the murmur becomes harsher and, besides, a faint diastolic murmur over the apex and in the third and fourth left intercostal spaces or in the second right intercostal space can appear). Moderate tachycardia is not pathognomonic, as it is often induced by pregnancy.

Chest radiograms reveal insignificant heart enlargement or changes peculiar to some forms of valvular heart disease (in recurrence of rheumatic carditis). Severe myocarditis can be accompanied by symptoms of pulmonary congestion.

The electrocardiogram may remain unchanged. When the disease has a typical course, the P-Q interval exceeds 0.2 s; P wave and QRS complex are altered; and ST segment depression and flattened, diphasic, or inverted T wave are observed. The changes recorded on the phonocardiogram are the same as those revealed by auscultation. Echocardiographic findings are those of impaired cardiac contractility.

The diagnostic value of "rheumatic" tests is rather relative.

In recent years no cases of heart failure during pregnancy were reported in patients with primary rheumatic carditis. In pregnant women with exacerbations of rheumatic valvular disease, rheumatic carditis is associated with a threat of heart failure.

7.1.1.2 Postinfective Myocarditis

This form of myocarditis, often observed in pregnancy after acute respiratory infections, is commonly believed to be viral (Hausen and Loch 1973). The course of postinfective myocarditis is relatively milder than that of rheumatic carditis, but in pregnant patients it is sometimes long-lasting and is accompanied by infrequent but stable premature beats, persisting sometimes after other manifestations of the disease have disappeared (Eliseev 1982). Infective myocarditis can develop some days after recovery from the respiratory infection.

The patients' complaints, as well as clinical and roentgenological patterns, are identical in postinfective myocarditis and in rheumatic carditis. Viral myocarditis is sometimes accompanied by pain in the skeletal muscles.

The P wave on the ECG is usually unchanged. Diphasic or inverted T wave is observed not only in standard limb but also in chest leads. ST segment is seldom changed. Sinus tachycardia and premature beats are often recorded. In some cases atrial fibrillation and other heart rhythm disturbances are observed. Transitory atrioventricular first- and second-degree blocks often develop and a left bundle branch block can be observed. Complete atrioventricular block is rare but can be the cause of sudden death.

In patients with myocarditis, especially of rheumatic origin, there is sometimes a risk of disease aggravation in pregnancy, though myocarditis itself seldom gives rise to heart failure in the absence of valvular heart disease (postinfective myocarditis can be accompanied by peripheral circulatory failure). If myocarditis is complicated by atrial fibrillation, thromboembolic complications are likely to develop. If severe myocarditis arises early in gestation, termination of pregnancy is indicated; in late pregnancy each such case is considered individually. In mild myocarditis and in the absence of serious coexisting diseases pregnancy is uneventful and not too strenuous for the cardiovascular system. On rare occasions, with the disease assuming an unfavorable course, myocarditis may transform into peripartal cardiomyopathy (Melvin et al. 1982).

7.1.2 Cardiomyopathies

7.1.2.1 Hypertrophic Obstructive Cardiomyopathy

Hypertrophic obstructive cardiomyopathy (idiopathic hypertrophic subaortic stenosis) has been more frequently diagnosed in recent years. Its etiology is unknown.

Familial forms of the disease are sometimes observed. The disease is characterized by marked asymmetrical hypertrophy of the ventricular septum and the adjacent left ventricular myocardium, reducing the size of the left ventricular cavity and disturbing the left ventricular function, especially in mid- and late systole, when contraction of hypertrophied myocardial regions creates an obstruction to left ventricular outflow. The degree of hypertrophy may increase with age. In addition, anomalous attachment (and hypertrophy) of mitral valve papillary muscles producing an anterior cusp forward motion is observed.

The hemodynamic sequelae of these morphological changes are the systolic pressure gradient across the outflow tract of the left ventricle (and in case of mitral cusp displacement, also mitral regurgitation) and disturbed ventricular diastolic relaxation.

The patients often complain of dyspnea on exertion, chest pain as in angina pectoris on effort, palpitation, weakness, and sometimes syncope. Palpation reveals a laterally displaced, enhanced (sometimes double) apical impulse. Auscultation reveals typical systolic murmur at the lower left sternal edge and at the heart apex, with the second heart sound audible (unlike in valvular aortic stenosis). The murmur can radiate to the carotids. The murmur is intensified in Valsalva's maneuver, with nitroglycerin administration, in the upright position, and is attenuated in response to pressor drugs and during squatting. In patients with affected mitral valve, systolic murmur of mitral regurgitation is heard at the heart apex. In marked subaortic stenosis the second sound is split and the third and fourth sounds might be audible. Arrhythmias are frequently observed.

Quite often changes in the peripheral arterial pulse are noted: it rapidly rises (in early systole), then attenuates (in mid-systole) and then one or two oscillations can be recorded before its diastolic collapse. The oscillations are clearly seen on the carotid pulse recordings. Systolic pressure (unlike in valvular stenosis) is not lowered and can sometimes even be elevated.

X-rays reveal left ventricular (sometimes also atrial) hypertrophy.

The electrocardiogram demonstrates signs of left ventricular hypertrophy, sometimes premature beats and atrial fibrillation, and, rarely, complete atrioventricular block. Very deep Q waves, ST segment elevation, P-R interval shortening, and left bundle branch block are observed.

Mesosystolic (beginning briefly after the first sound) murmur is recorded on the phonocardiogram; it may sometimes be diphasic. The later (with regard to the first sound) the murmur appears, the lesser the degree of stenosis. Other characteristic auscultatory signs are also recorded.

Interventricular septum thickening, abnormal forward motion of the anterior mitral cusp during systole, most clearly observed in Valsalva's maneuver and with amylnitrite inhalation, and reduction in the end-diastolic left ventricular volume are echocardiographically revealed.

Using heart catheterization and angiocardiography, the diagnosis is verified and the degree of obstruction to left ventricular outflow is determined.

The disease can be complicated by left ventricular failure. In some cases sudden death occurs even in asymptomatic patients, in whom the disease has not been recognized.

The increase in the cardiac output (and end-diastolic left ventricular volume) in pregnancy reduces the degree of obstruction in idiopathic hypertrophic subaortic stenosis; however, pulmonary vascular resistance (PVR) decrease has a reverse effect and the degree of obstruction remains unchanged. Pregnancy-induced increase in the inotropic cardiac function also has an unfavorable effect. In the second half of pregnancy, due to the compression of the inferior vena cava by the gravid uterus, venous return in the supine position is reduced, increasing in its turn the degree of dynamic obstruction. In the presence of concomitant mitral incompetence, pregnancy-induced hemodynamic changes may enhance regurgitation and even cause pulmonary edema. In addition, mitral regurgitation puts the patient at higher risk of subacute bacterial endocarditis (Kolibash et al. 1975). An adverse effect of expulsive efforts on the degree of obstruction can be compensated by the increase in the central blood volume, and finally rapid BV and left ventricular volume decrease can enhance the outflow tract obstruction. Though some cases have been reported (Brown et al. 1967; Shah and Sunderji 1985) when the condition of women with idiopathic hypertrophic subaortic stenosis worsened before and after labor, and some patients even died, an adequately managed pregnancy in women with mild and moderate obstruction is, as a rule, uneventful (Oakley et al. 1979; Evans-Jones 1983; Julian and Szekely 1985).

7.1.2.2 Peripartal Cardiomyopathy

The first report of a postpartal heart failure in a woman without a previous heart disease was published more than 130 years ago, and thereafter a number of such cases have been recorded in various countries of the world (mostly in Africa). And though more than a dozen possible etiological factors are suggested (deficient and disbalanced nutrition, preeclampsia, viral infections, drug hypersensitivity, endocrine disorders, genetic predisposition, immunological disorders, etc.), postpartal or, more correctly, peripartal cardiomyopathy is considered an individual nosological form, whose diagnostic criteria correspond to those of dilated (congestive) cardiomyopathy (Goodwin 1982). However, unlike the latter condition, peripartal cardiomyopathy may end in virtually complete recovery with the normalization of the patient's heart size (Julian and Szekely 1985). Pregnancy, possibly, only contributes to revealing the latent heart disease. The symptoms of the disease are often absent before pregnancy and labor, and can appear in the last trimester of pregnancy, within 3 months of the puerperium (most often) or, rarely, 5–6 months after labor (Demakis et al. 1971; Deeg 1983).

The etiology of the disease is as a rule impossible to determine. Moderate hypertrophy and marked dilatation of both ventricles (the left ventricle is more enlarged) are typical; mural thrombi are often observed in one or both ventricles. No changes in cardiac valves, coronary arteries, and pericardium are revealed (Meadows 1960; Julian and Szekely 1985). Diffuse degenerative alterations, myocytolysis and necrosis, as well as fibrosis foci are observed in the myocardium. Myocardial damage leads to a reduction in left ventricular contractility and a decrease in the ejection fraction.

Hemodynamic examinations reveal changes typical of heart failure: end-diastolic pressure elevation in the right ventricle, increased pulmonary artery and wedge pressure, in combination with a rise in pulmonary vascular resistance. Cardiac output is reduced but it may be normal in the early stages of the disease due to heart rate increase. Right ventricular and right atrial pressures are usually elevated.

The disease is more often detected in black women, in twin pregnancy, in multiparas over 30, and in patients with eclampsia. Heart failure develops in the last weeks of pregnancy, in the puerperium and very seldom before the third trimester of pregnancy (Szekely and Snaith 1974).

The patients complain of dyspnea and fatigue, sometimes of chest pain, coughing, and hemoptysis. Clinical examination reveals heart enlargement, manifestations of left and right ventricular failure, and arrhythmias; heart sounds are attenuated, the third and fourth heart sounds and systolic murmurs of mitral and tricuspid regurgitation are frequently heard. Roentgenological findings reveal heart enlargement and signs of pulmonary congestion. Life-threatening thromboembolism (more often in pulmonary than in systemic circulation) is frequent. Transitory moderate BP elevation can occur. The ECG commonly exhibits ST segment depression, flat, diphasic, and inverted T waves, a pattern of left ventricular hypertrophy, possibly mono- and multifocal premature beats, various arrhythmias, and atrioventricular and intraventricular conduction disturbances.

The echocardiogram shows left (and right) ventricular dilatation, left ventricular free wall hypokinesia, reduced velocity of circumferential myocardial fiber shortening, and sometimes evidence of mural thrombi.

The T-lymphocyte subpopulation pattern may be substantially changed (Sanderson et al. 1985).

The mortality rate is 15%–35%. One-third of the patients recover, and one-third retain clinical manifestations of cardiomegaly and electrocardiographic changes, but it is not always accompanied by worsening of the patients' condition (Meadows 1960). Spontaneous premature labor with fetal loss is noted in about 10% of pregnancies (Walsh et al. 1965). The overall perinatal mortality reaches 30%–34% (McAnulty et al. 1982; Hankins et al. 1985). The prognosis is satisfactory if heart enlargement promptly regresses (Deeg 1983; Levis 1983). The long-term prognosis for years ahead in patients with cardiomegaly is unfavorable. Repeated pregnancy in them should be avoided, as in women with persistent cardiomegaly it almost always causes the recurrence of the disease, resulting, as a rule, in the patient's death.

7.1.3 Specific Heart Muscle Diseases

The term specific heart muscle disease was proposed by the WHO Expert Committee on Myocardiopathies (World Health Organization 1984) instead of the previously used terms secondary cardiomyopathy and myocardosis. The term specific heart muscle disease signifies "heart muscle disease of known cause or associated with disorders of other systems" and includes metabolic (endocrine, deficiency, etc.), infective and general systemic diseases, heredofamilial abnormalities, and intoxications. Out of a variety of usually mild specific heart muscle diseases observed in pregnancy we shall be concerned only with those complicating severe thyrotoxicosis and anemia.

7.1.3.1 Thyrotoxic Heart Disease

In thyrotoxicosis the heart is affected due to the detrimental thyroxin effect and also due to enhanced sympathicoadrenal influences on the myocardium. In thyrotoxicosis the heart is damaged both because of intensification of general and cardiac metabolism.

As gestation is also accompanied by the intensification of metabolism, in severe thyrotoxicosis a hypertrophied heart works on the verge of decompensation.

The patients commonly complain of anxiety, weight loss, fatigability, palpitation, and poor heat tolerance. Examination reveals exophthalmos, finger tremor, and intensified carotid pulsation. Usually a slightly laterally displaced intensified apical impulse is palpated (in severe cases, the apical impulse displacement can become more marked, with its intensification disappearing). The heart sounds are initially loud; systolic murmur is heard over the heart base and apex, whereas with heart dilatation, the sounds become more muffled, atrial fibrillation is more frequently revealed, and the onset of heart failure is possible. The peripheral arterial pulse is rapid, large, full, and sometimes 90–120 beats/min. Systolic BP may be elevated and diastolic pressure may be reduced. Circulation time is shortened, sometimes even in the presence of heart failure.

Left heart enlargement, prominence of the aortic arch and pulmonary artery segment, as well as intensified pulsation of the heart and vessels are roentgenologically determined.

The electrocardiogram, besides sinus tachycardia, often exhibits atrial tachycardia and fibrillation paroxysms, increased P wave and QRS complex amplitude, and evidence of left ventricular hypertrophy. Less frequent are P-R and Q-T interval prolongation and the Wolff-Parkinson-White syndrome.

Echocardiography often reveals left ventricular hypertrophy and sometimes dilatation.

In severe thyrotoxic heart disease complicated by atrial fibrillation, pregnancy is contraindicated. Pregnancy should be terminated early, as the treatment of thyrotoxicosis in gestation is extremely difficult due to the drug toxicity and detrimental drug effect on the fetus (iodine drugs are ineffective in severe thyrotoxicosis, while propylthiouracil and thiamazol affect the fetus). Therapy with radioactive iodine and X-ray therapy are contraindicated in pregnancy. In moderate thyrotoxic heart disease surgical treatment of toxic goiter can prove effective, leading in the majority of cases to the regression of heart disease.

7.1.3.2 Anemic Heart Muscle Disease

Anemic heart disease can develop in pregnancy as a result of severe reduction in hemoglobin content. Anemia induces cardiac output increase and reduction in the peripheral vascular resistance that are already altered in pregnant women in the same direction. Marked anemia can be aggravated during pregnancy (gravid women frequently develop iron, B_{12}, and folic acid deficiency anemia).

The patients complain of weakness; they are pale and other manifestations of anemia are observed. The heart is enlarged (due to dilatation), tachycardia is usually present, and "anemic" murmurs over the heart are heard. BP is moderately lowered. Heart failure can develop. Termination of pregnancy is not necessary, as anemia responds well to treatment. Upon recovery from anemia the heart size normalizes and the murmurs and tachycardia disappear.

7.1.4 Myocardial Infarction and Sudden Death

Myocardial infarction is much less frequent in females than in males and occurs mostly in advanced age. Therefore, the disease was extremely rarely encountered in women of childbearing age. The infarction in this age group was generally caused by coronary artery anomalies, or early atherosclerotic alterations, mediated by hereditary hypercholesterolemias or severe diabetes mellitus. In the past decade due to the wide use of hormonal estrogen-containing drugs for long-term oral contraception the number of thromboembolic complications (including myocardial infarction) increased considerably (Motté et al. 1975; Mann et al. 1976; Jaillard 1983; Engel et al. 1983; Vessey et al. 1986). Estrogen administration produces lipid profile shifts, like those typical of atherosclerosis; BP elevation; and changes in blood coagulation, which are considered the risk factors of ischemic (coronary) heart disease. Thromboembolic complications are rather frequent in women with hyperlipidemia, arterial hypertension, and diabetes mellitus (Grand and Barillon 1976). They are more frequent in smoking women who take contraceptive pills. According to Rosenberg et al. (1983), regular smoking as a single risk factor increases the risk of myocardial infarction in young women fivefold. Naturally, chain smoking increases the risk to 10- to 13-fold and the combination of smoking with oral contraception heightens the risk of infarction 23-fold (Gerbert 1986). It must be noted that among 42 women who were oral contraceptive users and have survived a myocardial infarction 27 (64%) did not angiographically have coronary atherosclerosis (Engel et al. 1983). In cases when coronarography performed in the puerperium reveals no alterations in coronary arteries in women who had myocardial infarction during pregnancy, it can be retrospectively attributed to coronary spasm (Sasse 1975), or coronary thrombosis with subsequent spontaneous or drug-induced thrombolysis. Postmortem examinations of pregnant patients whose death was caused by myocardial infarction have demonstrated coronary atherosclerosis, coronary artery thrombosis, and sometimes coronary aneurysm or intramural hematoma (Hankins et al. 1985).

According to Ginz (1970), the incidence of myocardial infarction in pregnancy and in the puerperium is 1/10000 labors, and myocardial infarction mortality accounts for 28%; according to summarized data of Hankins et al. (1985), it reaches 37%. The mortality rate is higher when myocardial infarction develops near term, when labor starts earlier than 2 weeks after the onset of myocardial infarction and in reinfarctions. Myocardial infarction occurs mostly in the third trimester of pregnancy and in the postpartal pariod; it is less frequent in the first trimester of pregnancy (the outcome in this case is more favorable) and during labor. Cases of myocardial reinfarction before (Hankins et al. 1985) and after labor (Cohen et al. 1983) have been reported. Neonatal mortality ranges according to different data from 28% to 52%.

Some peculiarities are observed in postpartal myocardial infarction (occurring within the first 2 weeks after labor). It is more frequent in young primiparas who had preeclampsia. In some of these patients coronary artery atherosclerosis (usually one artery is affected) and coronary thromboembolism are detected, while in other patients the vessels seem unchanged and myocardial infarction is probably caused by coronary spasm. In some cases postpartal myocardial infarction results from coronary artery dissection (Shaver et al. 1978), presumably associated with the rupture of the intima and hemorrhage in the media (or with vasa vasorum rupture in the media) due to great strain during labor. In the majority of cases coronary artery dissection is the cause of sudden death.

Sudden death of women in pregnancy and the puerperium is quite rare. Cardiomyopathies, aortic stenosis, pulmonary hypertension and embolism, complete atrioventricular block, ventricular fibrillation, atrial myxoma, and isolated periarteritis with coronary artery thrombosis may be the cause of sudden death. This periarteritis of unknown etiology may, in some cases, be the cause of coronary artery dissection or the onset of aneurysm (Ahronheim 1977).

The diagnosis of myocardial infarction in pregnant women is not easy, though sometimes a typical clinical pattern, great emotional strain preceding a persistent pain attack, and characteristic changes on the ECG facilitate the diagnosis (Dementyeva et al. 1975; Cohen et al. 1983; Bornstein et al. 1984).

Myocardial infarction in pregnancy is often complicated by pulmonary edema.

In typical cases the main complaint is intensive compressing (or any other) retrosternal pain often radiating to the left arm or shoulder (or broader) lasting for 20 to 30 min and not responding to nitroglycerin. The nature and radiation of pain may not be typical. Physical examination reveals skin pallor and enhanced sweating. On day 2 of the disease a rise in body temperature is quite usual.

Auscultation reveals attenuated first heart sound, sometimes protodiastolic and presystolic gallop (the appearance of the third and fourth heart sounds) and systolic murmur over the heart apex, as well as heart rhythm disturbances. BP during pain attack rises and may then fall below the normal level.

The main electrocardiographic manifestation of myocardial infarction is the appearance of a wide and deep Q wave, and the earliest sign is ST segment elevation above the isoelectrical line (in leads recording electrical events in the unaffected myocardial area discordant ST segment depression is observed). T wave merges with the elevated ST segment, inverted deep peaked T wave forming 3–5 days later.

The elevated erythrocyte sedimentation rate and leukocytosis typical of infarction, as well as increased lactate dehydrogenase serum activity during pregnancy, are of no diagnostic value, while increased activity of creatine phosphokinase and especially its MB isoenzyme and aspartate aminotransferase retain their diagnostic value; this holds true for the rise in blood and urine myoglobin content in the extrapartal period.

Previous myocardial infarction probably does not constitute a threat for pregnant women (Murnaghan 1982), though some such patients do occasionally die. Acute myocardial infarction exposes pregnant women to a considerable risk, especially when it develops 12 weeks before or during labor. However, even in such cases the outcome is sometimes favorable.

Pregnancy should be avoided in women who survived myocardial infarction. Termination of pregnancy in the acute period of the infarction is associated with extremely high risk and should be avoided; later on adequate management of pregnancy and labor seems more advisable.

7.2 Diseases of the Endocardium

7.2.1 Subacute Bacterial Endocarditis

The microorganisms causing the disease are streptococci or staphylococci in 90% of cases. The disease is characterized by vegetations (consisting of fibrin, platelets, polynuclear white blood cells) of different size and shape appearing on the valvular cusps; they can spread to the chordae tendineae and endocardial lining of the heart chambers. The mitral valve is affected in 80%, the aortic valve in 60%, and both valves in 40% of cases. Microinfarctions often ensue due to microembolism of intramyocardial branches of the coronary arteries. Subacute bacterial endocarditis usually affects altered (like in acquired or congenital valvular heart disease) heart valves, as well as septal defects. Pregnancy is one of the predisposing factors, especially in the presence of infectious foci.

The disease starts with a slight fever, fatigue, and unclear muscular and articular pain. More seldom its first manifestation is cerebral embolism. Physical examination reveals petechiae on the skin, conjunctiva, and mucous membranes. Later the skin acquires a pale "earthy-yellowish" tint. The tourniquet test reveals increased capillary permeability and microvessel fragility.

Heart changes can be manifested in the murmur appearing over a formerly unaffected valve or sometimes in the altered nature of the murmur (appearance of a new organic murmur). Pronounced murmur changes are linked with the rupture of chordae tendineae or valvular cusp perforation, leading to dramatic increase in regurgitation, and can be accompanied by promt development of heart failure which usually appears later in patients with delayed or inadequate treatment. The electrocardiogram can record atrioventricular block (usually low degree) and atrial fibrillation, which is more often caused by rheumatic valvular heart disease.

Subacute bacterial endocarditis is characterized by embolisms in all the organs and tissues. Cerebral embolism constitutes the major threat though it is not usually fatal. The onset of meningitis (in this disease) is apparently caused by cerebral microembolisms (McComb et al. 1982). Embolisms of the spleen (followed by spleen infarction) and renal vessels and intramyocardial branches of the coronary vessels are most frequent. With the right heart chambers affected, pulmonary embolism and infarction, pneumonia, and abscess develop; the onset of pneumothorax is possible (Collins et al. 1985). Focal glomerulonephritis and renal infarctions are infrequent. Anemia is first normochromic and then hypochromic, the erythrocyte sedimentation rate is increased, some patients reveal moderate leukocytosis, and the number of monocytes in the peripheral blood is often elevated. The result of blood cultures can prove essential; however, they are sometimes falsely negative.

In recent years the course of the disease has changed (some manifestations may be absent), with the early period often latent. The timely diagnosis of subacute bacterial endocarditis in pregnancy is sometimes difficult, as subfebrile temperature, a higher erythrocyte sedimentation rate, moderate leukocytosis, and hypochromic anemia may be pregnancy-induced. Therefore, undetected endocarditis is probably relatively often revealed during postmortem examinations of women who died of heart failure during pregnancy and in the puerperium. Due to preventive measures (elimination of the infectious foci, asepticism), the incidence of bacterial endocarditis in pregnancy and the mortality rate have greatly decreased. At present, a new population of patients with subacute bacterial endocarditis has appeared — patients with prosthetic cardiac valves. Such patients sometimes get pregnant (Zimmerman and Shotan 1984). In such cases, the infective agent is not *Staphyloccocus aureus* or *Streptococcus viridans*, but uncommon microorganisms, making the treatment rather difficult.

Severe subacute bacterial endocarditis refractory to therapy with antibiotics is associated with poor prognosis and, therefore, in such cases pregnancy should be terminated early. In mild forms of the disease and successful treatment pregnancy can be preserved. Thromboembolic complications may be the reason for the termination of pregnancy, which exposes the woman to a certain risk (Szekely and Snaith 1974). Pregnancy in women who recovered after subacute bacterial endocarditis is uneventful in the majority of cases; however, in severe valvular heart disease heart failure can ensue. Pregnancy is allowed no sooner than 6–12 months after recovery from subacute bacterial endocarditis.

7.3 Diseases of the Pericardium

Acute isolated pericarditis is extremely rare in pregnancy (Probst and Mier 1963; Deeg 1983). Pregnancy is somewhat more frequent in patients with constrictive pericarditis; the disease either antedates or first appears during gestation (Krausz et al. 1978).

7.3.1 Acute Pericarditis

Acute pericarditis can arise after upper respiratory (often viral) infection, in the presence of connective tissue diseases and other disorders, but is most often idiopathic (benign or nonspecific).

Patients complain of sudden persistent retrosternal pain, sometimes radiating into the neck or the left arm (which is similar to pain typical of myocardial infarction; however, in pericarditis the pain is stronger on deep inspiration and slightly attenuates in the sitting-stooping position). At the early stage three- or two-component pericardial friction rub may be audible. Some days later retrosternal pain and pericardial friction rub usually disappear due to pericardial effusion accumulation. Very rapid pericardial effusion accumulation can give rise to cardiac tamponade with venous pressure elevation, arterial pressure fall, syncope, and threat of sudden death. Body temperature is usually elevated. Tachycardia is present and paroxysms of atrial flutter or fibrillation sometimes occur.

At the early stage of the disease the electrocardiogram records ST segment depression in all three (sometimes only two) standard limb leads and in most chest leads. In several days ST segment returns to baseline and inverted T waves appear. Echocardiography reveals the presence of pericardial effusion.

7.3.2 Constrictive Pericarditis

The etiology of the disease is difficult to establish. Constrictive pericarditis is characterized by fibrous degeneration of the pericardium often accompanied by calcification. The pericardium is often joined with the epicardium by adhesions and scars, placing the heart into the rigid membrane. The hemodynamic sequela is ventricular relaxation disturbance in mid- and late diastole, resulting in a dramatic end-diastolic pressure elevation and reduced venous inflow. Stroke volume decreases and cardiac output is maintained at near-normal level due to heart rate increase. Pregnancy-induced changes have diverse effects: the effect of high preload, enhanced inotropism, and chronotropism is positive, while the effect of peripheral vasodilatation is negative (Sullivan and Ramanathan 1985).

There are usually no data on previous acute pericarditis in history. Sometimes, there is reference to tuberculosis, rheumatic fever, respiratory infections, chest trauma, or signs of systemic lupus erythematosus.

The early stage of the disease is latent. Gradually weakness, fatigability, dyspnea, coughing, and vague pains in the chest, feet, and ankles swelling appear and progress. The advanced stage of the disease is characterized by right ventricular failure: hepatomegaly, ascites, and edema of the legs. Left ventricular failure is less prominent and manifests mainly on exertion. Physical examination reveals neck vein distension on inspiration, as well as systolic retraction of the heart apex and left parasternal and sternal areas.

Heart sounds are either normal or slightly attenuated, the second heart sound is split on inspiration, and the third heart sound can be heard. BP is usually normal, and arterial pulse pressure can be lowered. Sometimes pulse wave decrease during inspiration is noted. Venous pressure rises. Circulation time is increased.

Radiographic findings reveal a moderate heart enlargement in almost 50% of the cases (Silber and Katz 1975), with heart pulsation usually attenuated and lung fields clear. Pericardium calcification is often observed, and pericardial effusion (usually at one side of the pericardial cavity) is revealed in some cases.

The electrocardiogram demonstrates a marked reduction in ventricular complex voltage, often broadened and notched P wave, T wave flattening or inversion, atrial fibrillation, and sometimes flutter.

Blood volume increase in pregnancy is accompanied by further venous pressure elevation resulting in severe heart failure that may require surgical intervention during pregnancy. Pregnancy in women who recovered after pericardectomy can be uneventful (Mendelson 1969; Vanina 1971), especially more than 1 year after surgery.

Constrictive pericarditis should be regarded as a contraindication for pregnancy, if it has already occurred, termination of pregnancy is considered individually in each case, depending on the presence or absence of heart failure. Pericardectomy should be performed in the prepregnancy period.

7.3.3 Pericardial Cysts

Pericardial cysts are included in the cardiac pseudotumors. Usually, they are thin-walled formations fixed to the pericardium. They may be both congenital and acquired (blunt heart traumas, echinoccocosis), and when the cyst is connected with the pericardium it is considered a pericardial diverticula. Pericardial cysts are usually located in the cardiophrenic angle (more often right anterior), can be pedunculated, and change their position and shape with change in body posture.

The patients may be asymptomatic, although, sometimes they complain of recurrent weak pain in the heart area, or retrosternal pain that can occur independent of exertion. No auscultatory or electrocardiographic changes are observed. Pericardial cysts in pregnant women can be detected echocardiographically (Demidov and Fuks 1976) and roentgenologically. Spontaneous pericardial cyst ruptures are rare; no other complications are observed. Pericardial cysts are not a contraindication for pregnancy and labor. They are to be differentiated from disorders requiring surgical interventions: subdiaphragmal abscess, heart tumor, ventricular aneurysm, and hiatal hernia.

7.4 Uncommon Heart Diseases

7.4.1 Heart Tumors

Heart tumors are infrequent and rarely detectable intravitally, in part due to the similarity of their clinical manifestations to signs of other more common heart diseases, as heart tumors cause the same hemodynamic changes, heart shape alterations, rhythm disturbances, and embolism. In right atrial myxoma, for instance, signs of constrictive pericarditis, tricuspid stenosis or regurgitation, and pulmonary vascular thromboembolism are observed, while left atrial myxoma is often characterized by signs of mitral stenosis; and sometimes systemic embolism can arise. Right ventricular tumors can be mistaken for pulmonary artery stenosis and can cause pulmonic or tricuspid valvular incompetence. Left ventricular tumors can be erroneously diagnosed as subaortic or valvular aortic stenosis and when they cause local left ventricular prominence, the roentgenological pattern of ventricular aneurysm is observed.

7.4.1.1 Atrial Myxoma

The most common intracavitary primary heart tumor is atrial myxoma. It is usually located in the left and sometimes right atrium, bilateral myxomas being quite rare. The tumor is usually pedunculated and is fixed near the fossa ovalis area. It predominates in females. Large myxomas can almost fill the whole atrial cavity. The long peduncle enables the tumor to migrate from the atrium into the ventricle and back, in some cases obstructing the atrioventricular valve orifice.

Auscultation can reveal low-frequency mid-diastolic murmur without presystolic intensification or sometimes systolic murmur. The first heart sound is usually accentuated. With alterations in the body position both auscultatory and phonocardiographic manifestations of atrial myxoma can change in nature and intensity. Small myxomas can be asymptomatic. Atrial myxoma can be accompanied by embolism, pulmonary hypertension, progressive valvular dysfunction leading to severe heart failure, heart rhythm disturbances, syncope, and even sudden death. Accurate diagnosis (by echo- and angiocardiography) should be followed by urgent surgery that can be a success in pregnancy as well (Casarotto et al. 1979).

8 Heart Rhythm and Conduction Disturbances in Pregnancy

Heart rhythm disturbances in gestation are more often associated with valvular heart disease; however, they may also be observed in the absence of organic heart lesions. They are usually: sinus arrhythmia, occasional atrial or ventricular premature beats (sometimes even bigeminy and trigeminy), in some cases wandering pacemaker, atrioventricular junctional rhythm, and sinoatrial block. These arrhythmias do not cause hemodynamic disturbances and are, together with sinus tachycardia, frequently recorded on the ECG during labor. Patients with rheumatic valvular heart disease, along with the above heart rhythm and conduction disorders, reveal other arrhythmias and blocks; some of them markedly affect hemodynamics, can promote embolism, or sometimes constitute a major life threat. The prognosis is poor in atrial fibrillation, paroxysmal ventricular tachycardia, and complete heart block. Some arrhythmias and blocks are asymptomatic and can be revealed only by ECG recordings.

8.1 Cardiac Arrhythmias

8.1.1 Sinus Arrhythmia

Sinus arrhythmia is usually respiratory: heart rate increases on inspiration and decreases on expiration. P-P intervals of various duration are recorded on the ECG.

8.1.2 Wandering Pacemaker

Wandering pacemaker usually manifests in to-and-fro shifts of pacemaking activity between sinus and atrioventricular nodes. P waves of varying contours and P-Q intervals of varying duration are recorded on the ECG. This heart rhythm disorder is, like sinus arrhythmia, asymptomatic, and has no effect on hemodynamics, and the course of pregnancy and delivery.

8.1.3 Atrioventricular Junctional (Nodal) Rhythm

Atrioventricular junctional rhythm is characterized by AV pacemaker control over both ventricles and atria. It can result from depression in sinus node activity, sinoatrial blocks, or enhanced AV nodal automaticity. The ECG exhibits a negative P wave which may antecede or follow the QRS complex or may be lost within this complex. AV junctional rhythm arises infrequently and in the absence of organic cardiac lesions has no effect on pregnancy and labor.

8.1.4 Premature Beats

Premature beats occur due to impulse originating from the ectopic center or due to reentry mechanism. They can accompany a number of heart diseases and can occur in digitalis overdose and toxicity but they rather often result from autonomic nervous system dysfunction, reflectory influences from other internal organs, strong tea or coffee consumption, and emotional strain. Premature beats either are asymptomatic or are felt as thumping in the chest or heart stopping (sometimes both). Frequent premature beats cause cardiac output and coronary blood flow decrease, possibly leading to syncope or anginal attacks. Coupled and multifocal premature beats, as well as frequent premature beats, in pregnant women with mitral stenosis can antecede atrial fibrillation. In myocardial infarction early multifocal and coupled premature beats can presage paroxysms of ventricular tachycardia or ventricular fibrillation. The first sound of premature beats is usually accentuated, and premature beats are followed by a compensatory pause which is also revealed during peripheral pulse palpation.

The ECG in patients with atrial premature beats reveals deformed P waves located nearer than usual to the unaltered QRS complex. In ventricular premature beats P waves are absent, and QRS complexes are widened and deformed.

Occasional premature beats are clinically insignificant during pregnancy. Somewhat more frequent premature beats due to emotional strain or autonomic nervous system disorders do not pose an additional risk to pregnant women; however, they require therapy. Frequent and life-threatening premature beats should be treated and their cause should be established. The appearance of multifocal premature beats near term or in the puerperium can be a sign of peripartal cardiomyopathy. In marked extrasystolia termination of pregnancy is not indicated, if there is no severe heart disease.

8.1.5 Sinus Tachycardia

Sinus tachycardia is a regular cardiac rhythm of more than 90–100 beats/min. It can occur during physical exertion and emotional stress, fever, thyrotoxicosis, and marked anemia. It is detectable in many heart diseases and can be a manifestation of heart failure. The hemodynamic sequela of tachycardia is decreased cardiac output.

Tachycardia may be accompanied by a sense of palpitation. The contour and direction of atrial and ventricular complexes on the ECG are unaltered, and R-R intervals are shortened.

The significance of sinus tachycardia in pregnancy is determined by its cause, and the treatment should be aimed at eliminating this cause.

8.1.6 Paroxysmal Tachycardia

Paroxysmal tachycardia — attacks of acceleration in regular cardiac contractions to 100–200/min — can occur in the absence of organic heart disease, but is more often one of the manifestations of heart disease, thyrotoxicosis, infectious diseases, and digitalis intoxication; in rheumatic mitral valve disease atrial and ventricular tachycardia can sometimes presage atrial and ventricular fibrillation, respectively. The hemodynamic effect on the heart is unfavorable, especially with frequent and prolonged paroxysms. The appearance of frequent paroxysms of supraventricular tachycardia near term, during labor, and in the puerperium is associated with a certain risk.

Patients complain of sudden palpitation, sometimes accompanied by chest pain, dizziness, and enhanced sweating. Abundant urination at the end of the attack is quite often observed. Inspection may reveal vigorous carotid artery pulsation. The intervals between the first and second heart sounds become identical, the first heart sound is intensified, the second heart sound is faint, systolic BP decreases, and diastolic BP increases. The pulse is small and weak. A prolonged attack can be complicated by coronary insufficiency or heart failure.

In atrial paroxysmal tachycardia P waves are slightly deformed, they can sometimes be inverted and lost in the preceding T waves, and QRS complexes are intact. In ventricular paroxysmal tachycardia P waves are often undiscernable, and QRS complexes are widened and bizarre.

The incidence of atrial paroxysmal tachycardia attacks increases in gestation, in all the patients but for those with the Wolff-Parkinson-White syndrome (Hausen and Loch 1973). And if this does not seem significant in healthy women, in patients with rheumatic and congenital heart disease this can precipitate heart failure. Attacks of atrial paroxysmal tachycardia constitute a greater threat near term, during labor, and immediately after delivery. Paroxysmal ventricular tachycardia in pregnancy is infrequent. Paroxysms of tachycardia may sometimes first appear after delivery or in some cases occur only during pregnancy. Tachycardia paroxysms can be accompanied by increased uterine excitability. In marked rheumatic valvular heart disease prolonged tachycardia paroxysms can lead to pulmonary congestion or even pulmonary edema. And though the incidence of heart failure is relatively low (14%) the mortality rate in pregnant women can be high (5%) (Mendelson 1960). Thus, paroxysmal tachycardia in pregnant women with heart disease requires urgent and adequate therapy.

8.1.7 Atrial Fibrillation

Atrial fibrillation is caused by uncoordinated very frequent contractions of individual groups of atrial myofibers. High frequency and chaotic atrial contractions and fluctuations in atrioventricular conduction result in arrhythmic ventricular contractions of different intensity, their rate not exceeding 250/min. Atrial flutter is characterized by high-frequency (200–300/min) atrial contractions; every second, third, or fourth impulse in the absence of conduction variability is conducted to the ventricles. The absence of regular adequate atrial systoles is associated with decreased ventricular filling and reduced cardiac output in both atrial fibrillation and flutter.

Atrial fibrillation is most frequent in mitral stenosis. In pregnant women it can also accompany Ebstein's anomaly, digitalis intoxication, severe arterial hypertension, and thyrotoxicosis. Atrial fibrillation can be paroxysmal and sustained, tachy-, normo-, and bradysystolic.

Patients with tachysystolic atrial fibrillation complain of palpitation or thumping in the chest, dizziness, and sometimes chest pain. Subjective sensations are most pronounced during paroxysms of tachysystolic fibrillation, while bradysystolic fibrillation is better tolerated. In atrial fibrillation the intensity of the first and second heart sounds varies from cycle to cycle. When atrial fibrillation arises in patients with mitral stenosis presystolic murmur disappears. The pulse is arrhythmic, of varying filling. In tachysystolic fibrillation the number of peripheral arterial impulses is less than the number of cardiac contractions (pulse deficit). Instead of P waves the ECG records multiple fibrillatory waves of varying width and amplitude (in atrial flutter the waves are regular and homogeneous); ventricular complexes in tachysystolic atrial fibrillation are frequent and irregular (in atrial flutter ventricular complexes can occur regularly following every two to four atrial waves, or can sometimes be irregular).

Atrial fibrillation is threatened with thromboembolism and its tachysystolic form precipitates the onset or aggravation of cardiac failure.

Atrial fibrillation is the most frequent heart rhythm disturbance in pregnant women with heart disease; in rare cases it can be idopathic (of unknown etiology). As this arrhythmia has an adverse effect on hemodynamics and is associated with a risk of complications, its appearance during pregnancy poses a serious problem for it can increase maternal and fetal mortality. According to Szekely and Snaith (1974), atrial fibrillation first appears in pregnancy in 3.2% of patients with rheumatic valvular heart disease, who had sinus rhythm in the prepregnancy period. Atrial fibrillation can develop after the 4th month of pregnancy, when BV increase approaches its peak, which may probably cause distension of the left atrium. Such pregnant women become exposed to a particularly high risk of heart failure and thromboembolic complications (usually pulmonary artery embolism) soon after the onset of arrhythmias. However, modern preventive measures and treatment of these complications considerably decrease the maternal and fetal mortality rate in patients with atrial fibrillation, which a little more than 2 decades ago were 17% and 50%, respectively (Mendelson 1960). In recent years a decrease in the incidence of heart failure has also been noted among pregnant women with atrial fibrillation.

8.1.8 Wolff-Parkinson-White Syndrome

Wolff-Parkinson-White syndrome (WPW syndrome, preexcitation syndrome) is caused by anomalous atrioventricular conduction through accessory pathways (the James, Mahaim, Kent bundles; the latter may be left and right sided). The WPW syndrome is to a certain extent an electrocardiographic syndrome, including, in the presence of sinus rhythm, a short P-R interval with the QRS complex widening (from 0.12 s and more) due to the appearance of a so-called delta-wave (a small slurred additional upstroke in the initial part of the QRS complex). This type of ECG change is characteristic in the presence of the Kent bundles or combined James and Mahaim bundles. In the presence of only the Mahaim bundle, the P-R interval may be normal, while in the presence of only the James bundle the short P-R interval is accompanied by a normal QRS complex. ST segment depression below the isoelectrical line and diphasic or negative T wave can be recorded in cases with a widened positive QRS complex. The WPW syndrome can be congenital, namely in congenital heart disease, and predominates in women. The WPW syndrome can be temporarily removed by intravenous injection of 1 ml of 0.1% atropine solution. The impulse conduction through anomalous pathways can be downward and upward, and, therefore, a great number of patients with the WPW syndrome periodically experience arrhythmic attacks, more often those of paroxysmal tachycardia resulting from excitation wave circulation. However, a greater risk in atrial flutter and fibrillation is associated with transmission of atrial impulses along additional pathways (that possess an insufficiently long refractory period, as compared with the atrioventricular node), which can give rise to ventricular fibrillation and sudden death. The Wolff-Parkinson-White syndrome with attacks of paroxysmal reciprocating tachycardia or atrial fibrillation with high frequency of ventricular contractions can be observed in pregnancy (Gleicher et al. 1981); in pregnant patients with hypertrophic cardiomyopathy it may become the cause of death (Shah and Sunderji 1985).

Most patients with the WPW syndrome are asymptomatic, some of them having paroxysms of arrhythmia in history. Functional systolic murmur can be auscultated over the heart apex, vanishing with the disappearance of ECG manifestations of the syndrome; the first heart sound is accentuated (in cases of a normal QRS complex). Frequent and prolonged tachycardia paroxysms (that are quite rare) can lead to heart failure. In some cases ECG findings can simulate myocardial infarction (negative delta-waves) and bundle branch block.

In the absence of frequent and severe arrhythmia attacks pregnancy and labor are not threatened with cardiac complications. In frequent arrhythmia attacks pregnancy is contraindicated.

8.2 Conduction Disturbances

Heart block is a disturbance of impulse conduction at any level from the sinus node to the ventricles. The most common causes of heart blocks in women of childbearing age are rheumatic fever, nonrheumatic myocarditis, infectious diseases, syphilis, pronounced vagotonia, cardiac glycoside, quinidine, and procainamide overdosage. A complete atrioventricular block that dramatically diminishes cardiac output is of hemodynamic importance. The heart blocks are classified by the location of the conduction disturbance into sinoatrial, atrioventricular, and intraventricular. The block can be transient and permanent.

8.2.1 Sinoatrial Block

In sinoatrial block the impulse conduction between the sinus node and the atria is impaired, which results in an intermittent drop of single cardiac cycle (seldom two on end). This type of block is usually asymptomatic. Some patients have a feeling of missing a heart beat; when the dropped beats are frequent, the patients experience dizziness. Individual PQRST complexes with pauses equal to one (sometimes two) complexes can be absent on the ECG. Auscultation reveals periodic absence of heart sounds, while palpation of the radial artery demonstrates periodic absence of pulsation.

8.2.2 Atrioventricular Block

First-degree atrioventricular block is asymptomatic, except for attenuation or splitting of the first heart sound in many cases. The ECG exhibits fixed prolongation of the

P-Q interval by more than 0.2 s. In *type I (Mobitz I) second-degree AV block* each subsequent complex is characterized by progressive prolongation of the P-Q interval until the impulse conduction is blocked and only the atrial P wave is registered. Then the conduction is recovered, the sinus impulse is conducted to the ventricles at normal speed, and the cycle of conduction alterations is repeated. In *type II (Mobitz II) second-degree AV block*, the QRS complexes are dropped suddenly without prior P-Q lengthening. The patients may not have a feeling of "dropped beats"; however, they are either auscultated or palpated in the peripheral arteries. The first heart sound varies in intensity.

Patients with *complete atrioventricular block* (asynchronous independent regular or irregular atrial contractions and usually regular ventricular contractions) complain of dizziness and syncope, sometimes accompanied by convulsions (Adams-Stokes syndrome). Inspection may reveal rare abrupt pulsation (cannon wave) of the neck veins and their weak pulsation in pauses between irregular strong pulse waves (arising in simultaneous atrial and ventricular contractions). Auscultation detects rare (30–50 ventricular contractions/min) rhythmic heart beats with the first heart sound of varying intensity and cannon sound heard at irregular intervals (when atrial and ventricular contractions are simultaneous); sometimes weak atrial sounds are audible. Peripheral pulse is rhythmic, rare, and not accelerated on exertion. The ECG records completely independent electrical atrial and ventricular activity with relatively rare ventricular impulses. When the pacemaker is located in the AV junction the QRS complex is normal in shape, whereas when the pacemaker is located in the ventricle the QRS complex is somewhat widened and abnormal in shape.

The Adams-Stokes syndrome is caused by cerebral ischemia resulting from the absence of ventricular contractions for some seconds. It is manifested in pallor, dizziness, transient blindness and loss of consciousness, stertorous breathing, and sometimes also epileptiform convulsions, which are sometimes difficult to differentiate from true epileptic convulsions (the former are never accompanied by biting of the tongue) but which should be differentiated from eclamptic convulsions. Transitory cerebral ischemia is accompanied only by abrupt weakness or dizziness. The Adams-Stokes syndrome is noted in about 50% of patients with acquired complete heart block and less frequently in patients with congenital complete heart block.

8.2.3 Intraventricular Block

Patients with intraventricular block have conduction disturbances in one or in both AV bundle branches (or in one of the two fascicles of the left bundle branch). Such block causes no subjective disorders. The second heart sound is usually split owing to asynchronous ventricular contractions. In left AV bundle branch block the ECG exhibits widened QRS complex (its duration more than 0.12 s); in leads I, V_5, and V_6 the main wave of the QRS complex (R) is positive, the ST segment is depressed, and the T wave is negative; in leads III and V_{1-4} the main wave of the QRS complex is directed downward (S or QS), the ST segment is elevated, and the T wave is positive. In a right bundle-branch block the main wave of the widened QRS complex in leads I, V_{3-6} is negative, the ST segment is elevated, and the T wave is positive; opposite changes are registered in leads III, V_1, and V_2.

8.2.4 Heart Block in Pregnancy

The mere presence of sinoatrial block, first- or second-degree AV block, and intraventricular block does not seem threatening in pregnancy. The prognosis depends on the severity of the underlying disease. A complete heart block in active rheumatic fever can provoke severe heart failure and death of the pregnant woman (Mendelson 1960). In congenital complete heart block pregnancy is usually uneventful. Thus, according to Esscher (1981), 19 women with this type of conduction disturbance had 32 pregnancies and only 2 women had the Adams-Stokes attacks during 3 pregnancies. The heart rate in complete heart block can increase in the second half of pregnancy, and decrease during labor, possibly causing acute heart failure or the Adams-Stokes syndrome, if no preventive measures are performed. Pregnancy per se does not usually promote the first appearance or higher incidence of the Adams-Stokes syndrome in patients with complete heart block (Smirnova 1975). However, in patients with congenital complete heart block the Adams-Stokes syndrome may in some cases first appear during gestation (Sullivan and Ramanathan 1985). Nevertheless, a complete AV block with the rate of ventricular contractions less than 40/min and frequent Adams-Stokes attacks should be considered a contraindication for pregnancy. In such women pacemaker implantation is recommended (preferably before pregnancy).

8.2.5 Long Q-T Syndrome

A threatening conduction disturbance (both in the presence or absence of pregnancy) is a syndrome of the prolonged Q-T interval that may be a cause of syncope and sudden death due to ventricular fibrillation. This syndrome is observed in two hereditary diseases (the Jervell and Lange-Nielsen syndrome also manifested in congenital deafness and the Romano-Ward syndrome that is not accompanied by deafness) and poses a serious therapeutic problem (Zipes 1984). Clinical manifestation of conduction disturbances can first appear long after birth. Long Q-T syndrome can also be acquired, caused by various drugs, metabolic disorders, and heart disease. The patients can be effectively managed through uneventful pregnancy by β-blockers (Rubin et al. 1979); therapy with digitalis preparations is also possible (Wenger 1978).

8.3 Artificial Pacemaker and Pregnancy

The permissibility of pregnancy and labor in women with implanted artificial pacemakers constitutes a special problem. Preventive insertion of a transvenous temporary pacemaker electrode before labor made it possible to prevent or interrupt Adams-Stokes attacks; however, it is not always possible to avoid electrode displacement during labor. And, therefore, in recent years implantation of permanent artificial pacemakers is preferred. Women with an implanted pacemaker tolerate pregnancy well (Sullivan and Ramanathan 1985). Though a fixed-rate pacemaker does not allow the heart to react promptly to pregnancy-induced hemodynamic changes, it guarantees prevention of Adams-Stokes attacks. Programmable and demand pacemakers are preferable. There were doubts concerning the expediency of implantation of artificial pacemakers with isotope energy supply to women of childbearing age. The experience accumulated in Broussais's Hospital (Paris) has shown the safety and efficacy of a plutonium energy supply source: 20 women with congenital AV block gave birth to 25 healthy children. Irradiation from the source of energy was lower than the natural level of radioactivity (Laurens et al. 1983). This type of artificial pacemaker in pregnant women operated on for congenital heart disease was shown to be harmless for the fetus (Malbranche-Aupecle et al. 1985). If the severity of the underlying heart disease is not a contraindication for pregnancy in women with an implanted pacemaker, pregnancy does not hinder either the removal of electrode displacement or the change of the generator. If necessary, pacemakers can be implanted during pregnancy (Schaedel et al. 1977). In any case, the work of an artificial pacemaker in pregnant women should be constantly monitored. The most frequent disorder is a decrease in the rate of stimulating impulses; displacement of the endocardial electrode, skeletal muscle stimulation, and tissue irritation at the site of generator implantation are less frequent. In exacerbation of rheumatic carditis in pregnant women with implanted pacemakers, the decision to retain pregnancy should be made with consideration of the severity of the underlying valvular heart disease and myocardial functional state.

9 Pregnancy After Cardiac Surgery and Cardiac Surgery During Pregnancy

Modern advances in the field of palliative and radical cardiac surgery have allowed women with congenital heart disease and acquired valvular heart disease who were earlier unable to endure the hemodynamic burden of pregnancy and labor (or reach the childbearing age) to experience the joys of motherhood. From experience it follows that this new "population" of women who have undergone successful cardiac surgery should not be considered as having a normal cardiovascular system. It should be recognized that a previous disease or malformation could have led to changes in the heart muscle and pulmonary vascular bed, hardly completely reversible even after a successful surgical correction. Possible recurrence of rheumatic fever is not excluded. In addition, it is not always that the operation leads to perfect anatomical and physiological normalization of the cardiovascular system, and the residual defects should also be taken into consideration. For instance, even successful valvotomy that eliminates valve orifice stenosis fails to recover normal anatomical valvular structure and to guarantee the absence of restenosis in the future. Patients with prosthetic cardiac valves are often threatened with thromboembolic complications.

It is certainly preferable that the cardiac defect should be corrected prior to gestation. However, in cases when cardiac surgery is necessary (sometimes in life-threatening refractory pulmonary edema) it is performed during pregnancy, unless termination of pregnancy is thought preferable for the sake of the mother's life and health.

9.1 Pregnancy After Cardiac Surgery

At present in the whole world there are tens (probably hundreds) of thousands of women who have undergone cardiac surgery at childbearing age. The most numerous group among them comprises women after valvotomy. It was initially thought that pregnancy in postoperative cardiac patients was associated with a rather high incidence of complications (heart failure, thromboembolism) developing either during gestation or in the puerperium, which may sometimes prove fatal. A great number (7.5%–15%) of spontaneous abortions have been reported. However, in their comparative review Wallace et al. (1971) have established that the frequency of complications was virtually equal in the two subgroups of women after valvotomy (those who had pregnancy after the operation and those who did not). A tendency has even been noted toward a more favorable course of the disease in patients who had pregnancy and labor. However, it might be due to the fact that the women who made a decision to get pregnant were in a better condition.

Mlczoch et al. (1982) have reported a high proportion of surgically treated patients among pregnant women with congenital heart disease: out of 147 such women 88 had undergone surgery (53 — before and 35 — after pregnancy). Whittemore et al. (1982) compared the outcomes of 482 pregnancies in 233 women with congenital heart disease who had and had not undergone surgery. The outcomes depended on the functional class and were independent of previous surgery, except for patients with cyanotic heart disease. Unoperated women with cyanotic heart disease have given birth to only 42% of live children, all of them having a low birth weight; pregnancy in operated patients ended in 78% of live births. Congenital cardiac anomalies were found in 16.1% of children: surgery failed to diminish the incidence of congenital heart disease in children, which indicates the leading role of the genetic factor in this respect.

In women with congenital heart disease relief of cyanosis after surgery gives hope of uneventful pregnancy and labor in cases when the patients have good results of exercise testing. Successful correction of patent ductus arteriosus in childhood leads to complete recovery, and such pregnant women are considered apparently healthy. In other cases women after surgery for congenital heart disease or acquired valvular heart disease should be, irrespective of the results, considered cardiac patients. If such women conceive they should be managed through pregnancy and, if necessary, preventively treated.

The functional state of the myocardium determined by systolic time intervals improves but fails completely to normalize after valvotomy. In valvular heart disease cardiac performance in pregnancy can deteriorate even if valvotomy has been performed, especially when surgery has taken place during gestation and myocardial contractility has not fully recovered. Myocardial contractility can be also decreased in the puerperium, especially if surgery was performed in gestation or 7–9 years prior to it. The worsening of the condition is related to rheumatic fever recurrence, restenosis, limited functional reserve of the myocardium, and superimposed preeclampsia-eclampsia. Some surgically treated patients develop pulmonary hypertension (as a result of restenosis or a manifestation of inadequate valvotomy) in early pregnancy (Anichkova 1977). The most favorable time for conception is probably 1–2 years after the operation, when myocardial contractility has improved and restenosis has not yet usually developed. If pregnancy occurs sooner after surgery, it is somewhat more often complicated by heart failure. The functional results of the operation (assessed by exercise testing and hemodynamic values) are of paramount importance. The results are sometimes independent of the disease stage when surgical intervention took place. Auscultatory findings typical of heart disease can persist (or alter) but do not altogether disappear after surgery and cannot serve as a decisive factor in considering the problem of pregnancy and labor permissibility. In some cases pregnancy is possible after a successful operation on two or even three valves. Pregnancy can be contraindicated in patients after valvotomy if the operation was not sufficiently effective or in the case of recurrent rheumatic carditis, restenosis, pulmonary hypertension, atrial fibrillation, even early stages of heart failure, and torpid bacterial endocarditis.

9.2 Cardiac Surgery During Pregnancy

The first reports on the surgical correction of mitral stenosis during pregnancy date back to the 1950s (Brock 1952; Cooley and Chapman 1952). A great number of such operations have been performed since. At first cardiac surgery during pregnancy was performed when the indications were vital: in intractable pulmonary edema or progressive refractory congestive heart failure. At present the operations are often performed to improve the conditions of fetal development (Korolev et al. 1986). It is important to bear in mind that women who underwent cardiac surgery during pregnancy can have spontaneous abortion or premature labor in the postoperative period. There is no agreement as to the most appropriate time for cardiac surgery during gestation. Some authors are in favor of early interventions (Metcalfe and Ueland 1978); others believe the 20th–24th week of pregnancy to be the optimal time for surgery. If mitral valvotomy is performed in the 14th–26th week of gestation, when the placenta is already fully formed and hormonal changes are stabilized, enough time is left for heart adaptation to new circulatory conditions. Children of women operated in the 14th–26th week have greater birth weight than children of women operated later or neonates born by cesarean section to mothers with unoperated mitral stenosis (Korolev et al. 1986). The hemodynamic burden on the cardiovascular system is maximal in the 28th–32nd week of pregnancy, and, therefore, surgical interventions in this period should be avoided unless there are urgent indications. Cardiac surgery is also inadvisable during pregnancy in women with complicated obstetric history or current obstetric pathology. In life-threatening chronic congestive heart failure refractory to medical therapy cardiac surgery is not to be performed. In this case early, if possible, termination of pregnancy seems inevitable.

Judging from experience, even a much simpler operation, such as the ligation of patent ductus arteriosus performed during pregnancy can in some cases lead to spontaneous abortions and heart failure. Surgical correction of ventricular septal defect during pregnancy can cause complications, sometimes even fatal ones. Surgical correction of atrial septal defect during pregnancy is less risky for the mother; however, it, like every cardiopulmonary bypass surgery is associated with a certain risk for the fetus. Valvotomy in patients with aortic stenosis is usually uncomplicated in the absence of severe myocardial changes. However, surgery in patients with tetralogy of Fallot is associated with certain difficulties. Women who underwent this operation long before pregnancy often develop heart failure during subsequent pregnancies and there is a higher risk of premature labor and low birth weight of babies born at term. This can be attributed to the fact that the operation does not completely reinstate the normal anatomical status, and the cardiac muscle is not always functionally competent. Pregnancy after surgical correction of the coarctation of the aorta is usually uncomplicated. However, when the operation is performed during pregnancy, fatal anastomosis incompetence can ensue. In addition, after the removal of the coarctation of the aorta in some patients with concomitant congenital anomalies (bicuspid aortic valve, cerebral artery aneurysm), they may become a cause of complications in gestation. However minimal the operative risk, cardiac surgery should be avoided in pregnant women with congenital cardiac defects and acquired valvular heart disease. The operation is recommended in the prepregnancy period or even better before marriage. Taking into consideration the age of the pregnant woman, the form and severity of the heart disease, and possible unfavorable obstetric status, the physician should make individualized decisions on the possibility of retaining pregnancy or the necessity of pregnancy termination (preferably early) to give, if possible, the woman a chance to have the defect corrected in more favorable conditions.

The possibility of open heart surgery with extracorporeal circulation during pregnancy represents a complex problem. The first operation was successful; however, the child born at term had multiple malformations and soon died (Leyse et al. 1961). Initially, maternal and fetal mortality was 5% and 33%, respectively (Zitnik et al. 1969), some of the neonates having various malformations. Further on, technical advances and the decrease in the time of extracorporeal circulation, as well as the choice of the optimal time for surgery (after the 28th week of gestation), have brought about a decline in maternal and especially fetal mortality. Becker (1983) has reported that out of 68 pregnant women with mitral stenosis after open heart surgery only one woman died, with fetal mortality amounting to 20%. Nowadays a successful aorto-coronary bypass surgery (with the use of extracorporeal curculation) during the first half of pregnancy has been reported in a woman with left main coronary artery stenosis (Majdan et al. 1983). However, open heart surgery is preferable in non-pregnant patients, especially those with cyanotic congenital heart disease.

9.3 Pregnancy in Women with Prosthetic Cardiac Valves

Pregnancy in women with prosthetic cardiac valves poses a special problem. These women should be aware of the risk of pregnancy and of the limited opportunity to give birth to healthy children. It is still difficult to answer these questions definitely. At present the number of women with valvular prostheses who had one or sometimes two pregnancies has probably not yet reached 500. In the majority of cases pregnancy and labor were uneventful. However, there were cases of atrial fibrillation, heart failure, thromboembolism, maternal deaths, and more often fetal loss. According to summarized data, maternal mortality (almost exclusively in the postpartal period) was 6.3% and total fetal loss (spontaneous abortions, stillbirth, perinatal mortality) was 27% (Vanina and Smirnova 1978). The weight of 6% of neonates was below 2000 g, and 23% of the newborn showed retarded postnatal development. The incidence of spontaneous abortions and premature birth was 13%–32% (Deeg 1983). Stillbirths and early postnatal deaths were in most cases caused by hemorrhages associated with the use of coumarin-related anticoagulants during pregnancy. In addition, oral administration of anticoagulants (especially coumarin derivatives) in pregnant women is related to the increased risk of hemorrhages and spontaneous abortions (Sokolow and McIlroy 1981).

Palushchinskaya et al. (1981) have followed up 22 pregnant women with prosthetic cardiac valves. The use of indirect-acting anticoagulants (mainly phenindione) during pregnancy and in the puerperium did not always prevent thromboembolism in coronary and cerebral vessels (however, an adverse action of anticoagulants on the fetus was not observed in this study). In the antepartal period some patients had preeclampsia, progressive heart failure, and paroxysms of tachycardia; and in the postpartal period prosthesis functioning was sometimes disturbed, especially in multivalvular replacements. Mattoras et al. (1985) have reported 59 pregnancies in 48 women with valvular prostheses. Forty-four pregnancies were observed in women with cloth-covered metallic prostheses who had received anticoagulant therapy with coumarin derivatives and the rest occurred in women with biological prostheses who had not received anticoagulant therapy. In the first group one patient died; there were three cases of valve thrombosis, two cases of congestive heart failure, one case of puerperal hemorrhage, and increased incidence of premature delivery; retardation of the intrauterine fetal growth and low birth weight have been revealed and mild nasal hypoplasia has been observed in two children. The prognosis was worse in women over 30, 5 years after valve replacement, and with a history of thromboembolism and episodes of congestive heart failure. All the above findings once again illustrate the difficulties associated with the decision on the permissibility of pregnancy in women with prosthetic cardiac valves.

The functional results of valve replacement are not uniform. In most patients with aortic valve prosthesis myocardial contractility is close to normal, while in patients with mitral valve and multiple valve prostheses it is commonly disturbed; the patients of the latter two groups often develop atrial fibrillation. Pregnant women with prosthetic cardiac valves are exposed to the increased risk of subacute bacterial endocarditis and thromboembolic complications; there is also a threat of an adverse effect of anticoagulant therapy on the fetus. In addition, there is, irrespective of pregnancy, the risk of suture incompetence and prosthesis destruction.

Clinical manifestations of endocarditis caused by infectious lesions of any valve prosthesis are the same as in natural valve lesions. With normal functioning of a ball prosthesis "metallic" sounds that are not accompanied by any murmurs are auscultated. Fever, combined with the appearance of murmurs mediated by paravalvular blood leak, is indicative of endocarditis development. The murmur sometimes becomes heard some time after the onset of fever. The risk of endocarditis is particularly high in the intra- and postpartal periods, when transitory bacteremia is not uncommon. Endocarditis entails a number of complications. Bacterial colony (often yeast or fungi) growth on the valves can increase valvular orifice obstruction, leading to hemodynamic disturbances up to a gradual onset of heart failure. There is also a hazard of embolism with the colonies of microorganisms. The development of an abscess in the valvular ring area can entail prosthesis rejection. Adequate antiseptic and aseptic measures and preventive treatment make it possible, as a rule, to avoid the risk of subacute bacterial endocarditis.

Thrombus formation on the surface of the artificial valves is caused by the fact that prostheses are foreign bodies (in recent years not allografts but biological auto-, homo-, and xenografts that do not lead to thrombus formation are being used more extensively) and have a damaging effect on blood elements, causing the formation of platelet aggregates and fibrin depositions on the prosthetic valve surface. The incidence of thromboembolic complications in patients with valve prostheses ranges from 5% to 20%, being 17.9% in pregnant women (Vanina and Smirnova 1978). If prevention of bacterial endocarditis has no peculiarities in pregnancy, anticoagulant therapy during pregnancy should be performed with utmost care. In pregnant women with rigid valve prostheses withdrawal of anticoagulants received constantly after valve replacement leads to an increase in the incidence of systemic embolisms (Buxbaum et al. 1971), which may be attributed to the relative rise in the activity of the blood coagulation system during pregnancy. Pregnant women with prosthetic cardiac valves even on maintenance anticoagulant therapy do develop (more rarely however) thromboembolic complications: embolism in cerebral, pulmonary, and renal vessels, or sometimes valve prosthesis thrombosis. Thromboembolism in pregnant women on anticoagulant therapy is possibly related to inadequate drug doses and the lack of constant control over blood coagulation state. With the use of cloth-covered Starr-Edwards valves and biological prostheses that do not stimulate thrombus formation, there developed a trend to discontinue anticoagulant therapy in the remote post-operative period (Casanegra et al. 1975); however, even the use of modern valvular prostheses made of artificial materials does not guarantee the prevention of thrombo-embolic complications (Oakley and Doherty 1976). Thromboembolism is much rarer with the use of biological valvular prostheses. In patients with mitral valve prosthesis thromboembolic complications are more frequent than in patients with aortic valve prostheses probably due to the presence of atrial fibrillation and structural changes of the left atrium in patients with mitral disease.

Anticoagulant therapy, on the one hand, protects the pregnant woman from thromboembolic complications, but on the other hand, indirect-acting anticoagulants (coumarin and indanedione preparations) cross the placental barrier and pose a double risk for the fetus. Fetal loss in mothers who received coumarin derivatives before conception and in the first trimester of pregnancy significantly increases, as compared with fetal losses in women with prosthetic cardiac valves who did not receive such therapy (Buxbaum et al. 1971; Lutz et al. 1978) because of hemorrhagic complications in the fetus and intraplacental hemorrhages. The use of indirect-acting anticoagulants throughout pregnancy until term is threatened with the development of fetal hemorrhagic complications during vaginal delivery (but not during cesarean section). By term, blood coagulation in the fetus is normalized and perinatal hemorrhages do not develop if indirect-acting anticoagulants are discontinued a few days before labor. Heparin does not cross the placental barrier and, therefore, it is quite safe for the fetus; however, its constant parenteral administration is rather burdensome. Thus, heparin substitution for indirect-acting anticoagulants at least 2 weeks before term seems optimal. However, this is impossible in case of premature labor.

The second hazardous aspect of coumarin anticoagulant application is the threat of teratogenic effect on the fetus (chondrodysplasia, nasal hypoplasia, optic nerve atrophy, etc.). Indirect-acting indanedione anticoagulants (phenindione) seem safe in this respect, although their long-term administration exposes the mother to the risk of renal and hepatic failure. It should be noted that Oakley and Doherty (1976) have reported congenital malformations in two children whose mothers had valve replacements during pregnancy, one of the women receiving no anticoagulants. Malformations in children whose mothers received coumarin anticoagulants may sometimes, although very seldom, be observed as hereditary diseases (e.g., the Conradi-Hünermann syndrome), irrespective of the drug intake. A certain risk of teratogenic effect of coumarin derivatives cannot be discarded. The experience of phenindione use in 51 pregnant women proved to be encouraging, neither mothers nor children revealing any hemorrhagic complications (Vanina et al. 1979).

As there is a certain risk associated with the use of indirect-acting anticoagulants and frequent parenteral heparin administration is burdensome, attempts have been made to replace them by platelet aggregation inhibitors (acetylsalycilic acid, dipyrid-amole, and pentoxyphilline alone or in combinations) (Zucker and Peterson 1970;

Biale et al. 1980; Mok et al. 1985) or their combination with warfarin (Chesebro et al. 1983). The problem might be resolved by the use of porcine and human cadaver valves or fascia lata that possess no thrombogenic properties, and, therefore, require no constant anticoagulant therapy. However, the durability of biological valves is not always good, and, therefore, they sometimes require replacement. The close results of the operation are quite satisfactory. For instance, Denbow et al. (1983) have reported 13 pregnancies in 10 women with mitral and aortic homografts. Neither bleeding during labor nor teratogenic complications have ever been observed; this is attributed to the lack of necessity in anticoagulant therapy.

Preeclampsia-eclampsia in pregnant women with valve prostheses can considerably aggravate the patients' condition; however, it has not yet been established that preeclampsia-eclampsia occurs more often in this group of patients. In a number of cases, increased incidence of spontaneous abortions and premature labor is noted in women with prosthetic cardiac valves (Deeg 1983). The incidence of spontaneous abortions is very high in women who had a valve replacement during pregnancy (Vanina and Smirnova 1978).

The decision on the permissibility of pregnancy in women with prosthetic cardiac valves is individual in each case; it is always necessary to differentiate between the two extreme points: "pregnancy is inadmissible" and "pregnancy is not dangerous". The decision is based on the evaluation of the cardiac function, the results of surgical intervention, and the presence of concomitant diseases. The percentage of complications both in the mother and fetus being high during pregnancy in women with mechanical prosthetic cardiac valves, it seems preferable to recommend women who intend to undergo valve replacement first to give birth (in the absence of contraindications) and then to undergo surgery. After the operation, an optimal way of contraception should be selected. Pregnancy in patients with biological prosthetic cardiac valves seems permissible, because the danger associated with anticoagulant treatment is absent.

There are sporadic reports (Vanina 1971; Krauz et al. 1978) on the favorable course of pregnancy and labor in women after pericardectomy for constrictive pericarditis and after coronary artery bypass surgery (Majden et al. 1983).

10 Management of Pregnant Women with Heart Disease

The question of pregnancy permissibility (and safety for the mother and child) in women suffering from cardiovascular diseases should be discussed with a cardiologist (internist) long before pregnancy and preferably even before marriage. However, this is rather seldom achieved. If a women with heart disease does conceive and there are no indications for the termination of pregnancy, the patient should be put under constant supervision of a cardiologist (internist) with all the necessary preventive and therapeutic measures performed in order to avert (or reveal and remove) possible complications. Cardiovascular and urinary systems should be carefully examined not only during (and before), pregnancy but also after it, as they can be effected by pregnancy (in rare cases the onset of peripartal cardiomyopathy is possible; pre-eclampsia can lead to persistent renal disorders and become the cause of stable arterial hypertension).

10.1 General Principles of Management

The rational management and treatment of pregnant women with cardiovascular diseases is based on the accurate diagnosis with consideration of the disease etiology. In each case, the functional capacity of the myocardium should be assessed by hemodynamic examination and during graded exercise testing. In rheumatic valvular heart disease the degree of rheumatic process activity should be established (it should be determined three times — in the most likely periods of the disease relapse during gestation: in the first 3 and the last 2 months of pregnancy and also in the puerperium). The primary cardiological examinations should be performed in cardiological clinics or hospitals or in specialized obstetric units for pregnant patients with cardiovascular diseases, and in the absence of such hospitals and clinics, in specialized high-risk pregnancy units (or in obstetric antenatal clinics). Later on, the patient should be managed in obstetric (preferably specialized) clinics (hospitals) where she is to be examined by a team of specialists, necessarily including a cardiologist (internist).

Taking into consideration that the maximal hemodynamic burden arises in the 7th–8th months of gestation and during labor, pregnant women with cardiovascular diseases should be hospitalized at least three times. The first hospitalization should take place in the 8th–10th week of gestation for a more accurate diagnosis and to consider retention of pregnancy. Repeated planned hospitalizations should take place in the 28th–29th week of gestation (for examination of the patient's cardiovascular system and, if necessary, the support of the cardiac function in the period of maximal physiological hemodynamic changes) and in the 37th–38th week of gestation (to prepare the patient for labor and to select an optimal way of delivery). The patient should be admitted to hospital no later than the beginning of the 39th week of gestation. After delivery, women who have had rheumatic carditis recurrence during pregnancy should, in the absence of obstetric complications, be placed under medical care in a hospital for internal or cardiovascular diseases. With the onset of heart failure, rheumatic carditis relapse, the development of myocarditis and endocarditis of nonrheumatic etiology, atrial fibrillation, complete atrioventricular block, or signs of preeclampsia or marked anemia, the patient should by hospitalized any time during pregnancy.

As pregnancy is characterized by abrupt hemodynamic changes, pregnant women with cardiovascular diseases should undergo regular cardiological examinations every 2 weeks, and even more frequently by the end of the gestational period. In all cases the patient should be managed by a cardiologist (internist) and an obstetrician, who make a joint decision on the method of treatment, optimal way of delivery, or the necessity of termination of pregnancy. In hospital it is essential to detect and treat concomitant diseases (anemia, hyperthyroidism, urinary tract infections, etc.) and eliminate chronic infectious foci.

Whether the woman is allowed to retain pregnancy should be decided in the first 12 weeks of gestation. Termination of pregnancy is indicated in the presence of subacute bacterial endocarditis, severe rheumatic carditis, severe myocarditis, cardiomyopathy, severe mitral stenosis and mixed mitral valve disease with predominant stenosis, combination of mitral stenosis and aortic regurgitation, severe aortic valvular stenosis, marked tricuspid regurgitation, tricuspid stenosis, pulmonic valve stenosis, coarctation of the aorta, cyanotic congenital valvular heart disease, primary pulmonary hypertension, Eisenmenger's syndrome, Marfan's syndrome with significant alterations of the aortic root, cardiomegaly of any etiology, heart failure (NYHA functional class III–IV) arising in any congenital heart disease during the previous pregnancy, 1 year before the current pregnancy or in the first 12 weeks of gestation, atrial fibrillation, pulmonary hypertension in any form of congenital or acquired heart disease, congenital or acquired heart disease in combination with arterial hypertension, and chronic glomerulonephritis or thyrotoxicosis (indications for the termination of pregnancy in various forms of arterial hypertension and vascular disease are listed in the respective chapters). In the rest of the cases, the decision on early termination of pregnancy depends on the severity of the heart disease, functional state of the circulatory system, and degree of rheumatic process activity, if any. A decision on the necessity of late termination of pregnancy presents certain difficulties. In such cases, with the onset of heart failure or any intercurrent diseases, the woman should be hospitalized and subjected to thorough examination and adequate therapy. When active measures to relieve heart failure are ineffective and there are contraindications for cardiac surgery, the physician must decide on the termination of pregnancy at any time of gestation. Extraamniotic administration of saline or prostaglandin $F_{2\alpha}$ is absolutely prohibited in pregnant women with cardiovascular diseases. A more than 26-week pregnancy should be terminated by abdominal cesarean section. In promptly progressing refractory cardiac failure cesarean section is sometimes performed; however, it should be recognized that surgery per se (without medical therapy) does not relieve decompensation, but only promotes the drug effects. In some cases, conversely, cesarean section and prompt fetus extraction followed by uterine contraction, promoting blood redistribution, can cause acute heart failure. Therefore, in each case when the necessity of late termination of pregnancy arises, the cardiologist (internist) and the obstetrician should arrive at a common conclusion as to what is more risky: to terminate or to retain pregnancy. In some cases in the presence of heart failure, valvotomy in late pregnancy is sometimes safer and, therefore, more expedient than cesarean section in women with mitral stenosis.

Breast-feeding is usually allowed in women with cardiovascular diseases, but in pronounced heart failure lactation should be suppressed. In recent years, instead of tight bandaging of the mammary glands, bromocriptin has been administered orally, one tablet (2.5 mg) twice daily for 2 weeks. Estrogens are inadvisable, as there is a persistent risk of thrombophlebitis and pulmonary artery thromboembolism.

10.2 Regimen and Diet

The level of physical activity (which should be rather high in healthy pregnant women) is adjusted individually in each case. The activity of patients with mild to moderate myocardial and valvular changes (e.g., in mild mitral or aortic regurgitation) is to be somewhat limited, while in severe cardiovascular disorders hospitalization and strict bed rest are recommended. Rest and sleep in the left lateral position are advised to pregnant women with heart diseases characterized by limited preload (aortic valvular stenosis, coarctation of the aorta, hypertrophic obstructive cardiomyopathy, etc.). Since exertion increases an already elevated cardiac output, strenous, abrupt, and isometric load should be avoided. At the same time complex therapy, including graded physical exercise (used with regard to exercise tolerance) has a favorable effects on the condition of pregnant women suffering from rheumatic valvular heart disease and reduces the incidence of complications during pregnancy and labor (Kuzmenko 1980). Special physical exercise complexes can be applied even in respect to patients with heart failure. With the appearance of dyspnea or other symptoms of heart failure at an ordinary level of exercise, the patient should be hospitalized, as a life-threatening pulmonary edema can develop even in patients who were asymptomatic in the prepregnancy period, or may be induced by such factors (namely emotional overstrain) which earlier did not influence the state of the circulatory system. The patients are recommended to have 1 or 2 h rest in the daytime and sound sleep at night (sometimes it is achieved by giving them mild sedatives harmless for the fetus); the night's sleep should be 1 h longer than in the prepregnancy period. Bed rest is indicated in the last weeks before term, as heart failure and heart rhythm disturbances are less frequent and respond better to therapy in patients following a bed rest regimen.

Pregnant women with heart diseases may be more than normally susceptible to the effect of some environmental factors. The combination of heat and humidity (at home and at work) increases the hemodynamic burden and can, in conditions of unstable compensation, contribute to the development of heart failure. Work with any sources of ionizing radiation or in other occupationally hazardous conditions may have a detrimental effect on the fetus and aggravate the course of heart disease. Therefore, pregnant women with cardiovascular diseases should work in nonhazardous conditions at normal temperature and humidity. To avoid congestion in the leg veins, passive standing is not recommended (during walking and even limited movements of the legs muscular contractions ensure blood outflow from leg veins). It is advisable to avoid both excess bending of the knees while sitting and lying on one's back (it is preferable that the patient lies on her side while resting).

Since pregnant women rather often have respiratory infections, exerting an additional burden on the circulatory system, measures should be taken for their prevention, or early detection and treatment. Absolute abstention from smoking, which has become a "catching" habit with many young women, is essential in this respect. Smoking has been shown (Asmussen 1978, 1979) to reduce placental mass by 20%, to decrease the birth weight and size of the newborn by 10%, and to cause pathological changes in the basal membrane endothelium and umbilical artery and vein myocytes, which is indicative of possible intrauterine damage of other fetal vessels as well. One to two cigarettes a day cause a transitory BP rise in pregnant women (Biggs 1975), which is extremely undesirable, especially in preeclampsia. Smoking women have a higher incidence of spontaneous abortions in the first trimester of pregnancy, premature labor, and stillbirths. Perinatal mortality in offsping of smoking women is higher (Meyer and Tonascia 1977; Asmussen 1979) and the incidence of congenital anomalies in them, including congenital heart disease, is almost 1.5 times higher than in nonsmoking women. Children of smoking mothers remain physically and mentally retarded during the 1st year of life. A direct correlation has been established in pregnant women between the number of cigarettes per day and the risk of tumor development in their offspring. In the most exposed group it increases by 50%. A 100% higher risk of non-Hodgkin's lymphoma, acute lymphoblastic leukemia, and Wilm's tumor was observed (Stjerfeldt et al. 1986).

Urinary tract infections (namely pyelonephritis) seem no less frequent in pregnant women than respiratory infections. They form an undesirable infectious focus, especially in patients with heart diseases, and in those with acute pyelonephritis that, assuming a chronic form, can cause secondary arterial hypertension.

The woman's (especially the primigravida's) worries as to the course and outcome of pregnancy can lead to nervous overstrain that may have an adverse effect on the cardiovascular function and can aggravate the woman's condition. Considerable nervous strain can provoke pulmonary edema in pregnant and nonpregnant young women with mitral stenosis (Perloff 1984); anxiety can also be a cause of paroxysmal tachycardia and atrial fibrillation. In order to calm the patient, it is often sufficient to have a frank, reassuring talk with her. The physician should explain to her the specific features of pregnancy, labor, and puerperium with respect to her particular disease and condition and remove the fear in face of labor. Coordination between a cardiologist (internist) and an obstetrician is obligatory to avoid conflicting information and recommendations.

The patients' diet should be optimal and well balanced, but not excessive in calories, as it is not only sodium and water retention, frequent in pregnancy, but also obesity that increase the cardiovascular burden. Nutrition of pregnant women with cardiovascular diseases is based on diversified diets for patients with rheumatic valvular heart disease and those with heart failure (Samborskaya and Gutman 1984). The diets of patients with rheumatic valvular disease should contain increased amounts of high-value proteins, potassium, iron and vitamins C and B, somewhat decreased amounts of carbohydrates and considerably reduced amounts of salt. Women of medium size (155–165 cm) and weight (55–60 kg) should, in the first half of pregnancy, be kept on a diet containing 110–120 g proteins, 70–80 g fats, and 250–300 g carbohydrates, with an energy value of 10050–11300 kJ (or 2400–2700 kcal). In the second half of pregnancy the components should amount to 120–130 g, 80–90 g, and 300 to 350 g, respectively, with an energy consumption of 11750–12560 kJ (2700–3000 kcal). The energy value of a diet should be reduced by 1680 kJ (400 kcal) in short women of low weight, and increased by 840–1260 kJ (200–300 kcal) in tall women of considerable weight. In exacerbation of rheumatic fever, the protein and fat content should be temporarily reduced to 70–80 g and 200–250 g, respectively. Meals should be taken five to six times a day. Animal proteins should constitute about 50% of the total amount of proteins consumed. Complex carbohydrates are preferable (wholewheat bread, vegetables, cereals, fruit, berries); the amount of simple carbohydrates (sugar, cakes, etc.) is to be limited in the food of pregnant women. The daily diet should include 25–30 g vegetable oil. The food must be rich in vitamins, as the need for vitamins in pregnancy increases almost twofold. A diverse menu consisting of milk, cottage cheese, nonsalty brands of cheese, butter, meat, fish, liver, kidneys, eggs, beans and peas, buckwheat, oatmeal, potatoes, bread, yeast, vegetables, fruit, and berries supplies the pregnant woman with the necessary amount of vitamins. In some cases, the patients should also receive vitamin preparations. Sufficient calcium, magnesium, potassium, and iron consumption is essential in pregnancy. Salts of these metals are present in most of the above foodstuffs. In iron-deficiency anemias, iron-containing preparations are sometimes to be used. Water, salt, and animal fat consumption in pregnant women with cardiovascular diseases should be limited to 1000–1200 ml/day, 2–5 g/day, and 40 g/day, respectively. Fatty meat and fish, pickles, smoked fish and meat, chocolate, strong tea, and coffee should not be included in the pregnant woman's diet. To control body weight pregnant women should be weighed every day before breakfast. In water retention, moderate doses of diuretics should be given for short periods. In case a woman is predisposed to constipation, yogurt, boiled beet, prunes, and fresh plums or laxatives of vegetable origin are indicated.

Along with special physical exercise complexes (including breathing exercises), oxygen therapy, psychoprophylactic training, relaxation, and autogenic training are advisable.

In patients with congenital heart disease, nutrition, depending on the state of the cardiovascular system, can be ordinary, the same as in women with acquired heart disease, or modified, in the presence of heart failure. In the early stages of heart failure, protein and fat consumption as well as energy value are slightly decreased, water intake being reduced to 0.8 liters. In severe heart failure, the protein content in the diet is decreased to 60–80 g (two-thirds to be of animal origin), and fat, energy, and water content is limited to 50 g, 9210–10470 kJ (2200–2500 kcal), and 0.6 to 0.7 liters, respectively. A low-energy diet should be alternated with a high-energy diet (Samborskaya and Gutman 1984).

10.3 Treatment and Prophylaxis

The principles of medical management of pregnant women with congenital heart disease and other cardiovascular pathology do not differ from the management of nonpregnant patients with the corresponding diseases. However, therapy of pregnant women is also directed at attenuating the pregnancy-induced hemodynamic shifts. Medical therapy in pregnant women should be performed with consideration of its potential effects on the fetus.

In recent years 2%–3% of all newborns had congenital malformations. In such countries as France and the United Kingdom 20000–25000 children with congenital anomalies are born annually (Tuchmann-Duplessis 1975). The birth rate of children with congenital malformations might be even higher as many congenital anomalies (including cardiac anomalies) are detected months or years after birth. Though the increase in the percentage of children with congenital malformations can be, to a certain extent, related to an abrupt fall in infantile mortality from infectious diseases, it is most likely that an ever complicating environment plays, if not a predominant, then an essential role in this respect. Of the four basic groups of etiological determinants causing malformations — genetic, chromosomal, exogenous, and multifactorial — the latter two are of the greatest importance due to their predominance. Fetal malformations can occur in women working at chemical enterprises (production and processing of substances containing carbon disulfides, mercury, lead, arsenic, antimony, manganese, fluorine, cadmium, and some other elements) or at pharmaceutical plants. Even concentrations near maximum permissible levels are already dangerous, as many chemical substances can cross the placental barrier and accumulate in the fetus. The teratogenic effects of ionizing radiation in early pregnancy are common knowledge. Irradiation is most dangerous on the 18th–38th day after conception. Irradiation of the fetus later in pregnancy can lead to growth retardation or cause functional incompetence of the central nervous system (Rugh 1969). It should be noted that exposure of fetal gonads to small doses of ionizing radiation can mediate genetic disorders without causing malformations. Fluoroscopy should be avoided in the first trimester of pregnancy and in the gestational period in general, as the irradiation dose during fluoroscopy without electronic amplifier is about ten times higher than during roentgenographic examination.

Pesticides, herbicides, and fungicides constitute a serious hazard for pregnant women, not only those engaged in their production (pesticides, for instance, can penetrate many food products). The so-called food additives (for food preservation or the improvement of its appearance and taste), smoking, alcohol consumption, and some drugs (especially in early pregnancy) pose potential threats.

10.3.1 Drugs and Pregnancy

The detrimental effects of some drugs on the fetus cannot always be considered only as the result of exogenous factor influence. The interrelationships may be complex. The etiology of malformations may be multifactorial. Along with the exogenous factor effect, gene(s) sensitive to them can play an additional role. This fact can explain why the use of the same drug in different women in an identical dose and duration of administration and in the same period of pregnancy does not always end in the birth of offspring with malformations; in many cases mothers do give birth to normal children. Individual peculiarities in mothers with regard to absorption, metabolism, and excretion of different drugs seem essential.

An important question arises concerning the time when the risk of the damaging effect of drugs (and other exogenous factors) on the fetus is the greatest during pregnancy. It has been established that there are critical periods of fetal development, when the fetus is most sensitive to pathogenic effects of environmental factors. After blastocyst implantation into the decidua (on the 7–8th day after conception) organogenesis and placentation periods lasting 3–4 months commence. The critical phase in this period is the first 3–8 weeks (20–40 days for the heart). As different organs and systems are formed and developed at various periods, the damaging effect of environmental factors (for instance, that of some drugs) can become manifest with respect to this or that organ or system depending on when the exposure to it took place in gestation. Some damaging exogenous factors have tropism to certain organs. The notorious thalidomide (advertised in many countries of western Europe as a special soporific, antiemetic, and tranquilizing agent for pregnant women) has proved to be a universal teratogen, as its long-term application caused not only limb malformations but also anomalies of other organs. However, in some instances the drugs used in the same period during pregnancy may in different cases cause defects of different organs, i.e., these drugs are likely to possess polyfocal tropism.

In the first 6–8 weeks of gestation the physician should avoid the prescription of any drugs (except for life-threatening cases) and especially those whose detrimental effect on the fetus is common knowledge. In the first 3–4 months of pregnancy drug therapy should be performed with utmost caution. Later in pregnancy practically no embryotoxic and teratogenic drug effects are observed (Kirushchenkov 1978). It is only preparations with an androgenic effect that might cause signs of false male hermaphroditism in the female fetus. The risk of embryotoxic and teratogenic effect of drugs should not be overexaggerated, as the refusal to use them rationally can do harm to the health of the mother and her expected child. Most drugs used for the treatment of extragenital and obstetric pathology are harmless for the fetus.

A cardiologist (internist) and obstetrician often have to consider whether it is necessary, expedient, and safe to use antimicrobial drugs in pregnant women for the prevention of the recurrence of rheumatic fever and treatment of bacterial endocarditis and other infectious diseases. Various antibiotics cross the placenta at a different rate and in different amounts. Penicillin is rather fast to cross the placenta; it is harmless for the fetus, even at high doses. The same holds true for its long-acting analogues. Semisynthetic penicillins (ampicillin, oxacillin, dicloxacillin) also possess neither teratogenic nor embryotoxic properties (Kunz and Schreiner 1982; etc.). However, as ampicillin crosses the placenta in the greatest amount, its mean intramuscular single dose should not exceed 500 mg, to avoid possible development of nuclear jaundice in the fetus (Kirushchenkov 1978).

Short-term use of streptomycin at usual doses has no teratogenic or embryotoxic effects; however, in long-term application it may damage the fetal acoustic nerve. Therefore, its use should be avoided in pregnancy (Berglund et al. 1984).

Antibiotics-aminoglycosides (neomycin, vancomycin, kanamycin, gentamycin) are of limited application due to their nephro- and ototoxicity (Pepperell 1983), and it is preferable to avoid their use (Kunz and Schreiner 1982; Berglund et al. 1984; etc.).

Tetracyclines have no teratogenic effect according to some authors (Lauritzen 1985). However, other authors (Berglund et al. 1984; Zierler and Rotman 1985) report cases of their teratogenic action. However, their use after the 4th month of gestation can lead to brownish staining of milk teeth and multiple caries, while long-term use of the drug until late pregnancy can affect the color of the permanent teeth. Long-term tetracycline use may cause fetal growth retardation (Tuchmann-Duplessis 1975) due to its accumulation at high concentrations in bone calcification areas of the extremities (Kunz and Schreiner 1982; Berglund et al. 1984; etc.). Therefore, the tetracyclines should be avoided in pregnancy at least from the 4th month of gestation.

Chloramphenicol has no teratogenic effect but may cause a so-called gray syndrome in the newborn (the newborn's skin is of gray-cyanotic color due to peripheral vascular collapse; it vomits, is unable to drink, and has muscular hypotension and dyspnea) due to disturbances in the glucuronization process, as well as leukopenia and fetal hypoplastic anemia (Kirushchenkov 1978). Severe gray syndrome may lead to the newborn's death, but in cases of necessity the drug may be used until the 28th week of pregnancy (Kunz and Schreiner 1982).

Antibiotics of the cephalosporin group (cephaloridine, cephalexin, cephalozolin) possess no teratogenic or embryotoxic properties (Kunz and Schreiner 1982; Pepperell 1983, etc.); however, some authors (Mashkovsky 1984) do not recommend their use in the first months of pregnancy.

Erythromycin, ristocetin, and fusidate sodium pass through the placenta in limited quantities and have no adverse effect on the fetus (Kirushchenkov 1978). If need be, the following drugs, which possess no teratogenic properties can be used: clindamycin, lincomycin, oleandomycin, polymyxin, and colistin (Kunz and Schreiner 1982; Lauritzen 1985; etc.).

Sulfonamides easily cross the placenta, some of them causing facial bones and tooth pathology in the experiment. Cases of nuclear jaundice caused by nonconjugated bilirubin penetrating into the central nervous system tissues have been reported in the offspring of mothers treated with sulfonamides. Sulfonamides, possessing high binding capacity to blood plasma proteins, seem capable of displacing bilirubin from protein-binding sites, thus inducing toxic concentrations of free bilirubin in the blood plasma. It should be noted that sulfonamides might aggravate the course of isoimmunization (in Rh- and ABO-incompatibility) and enzyme deficit in glucose-6-phosphate-dehydrogenase deficiency (Baskin et al. 1980). If need be, sulfonamides (preferably not long acting) may be used (Kunz and Schreiner 1982) but not in the third trimester of pregnancy. Sulfonamides, for instance, have to be used in allergy to penicillin and other antibiotics.

Nitrofurantoin passes through the placenta, exhibits no teratogenic effect, but probably causes neonatal hemolysis and, therefore, its use in the third trimester of pregnancy is undesirable (Kunz and Schreiner 1982; Pepperell 1983; etc.).

Chloroquine, which refers to the group of quinolinic antimalarial agents, is at present used quite extensively for the treatment of lingering and recurrent rheumatic fever and some other collagenoses. As the drug affects histogenesis in the central nervous system and there are reports (Smith 1966) of deaf children born to mothers who received chloroquine during pregnancy, the drug is contraindicated in gestation, especially in the first trimester.

Glucocorticoids, used for the treatment of rheumatic fever and other collagenoses, were experimentally shown to cause different anomalies, though extremely rare in humans (cleft palate) occurring only with high drug doses. However, in the first trimester of pregnancy, glucocorticoids should be used only if unavoidable, as according to Serment and Ruf (1968), who followed up a great number of pregnant women receiving glucocorticoids in this period of gestation, 2.5% of newborns had congenital malformation and 2.8% of mothers had premature labor. Long-term use of large glucocorticoid doses can give rise to adrenal cortex atrophy in the fetus, sometimes manifested in acute adrenal failure of the newborn, which requires the injection of increasing corticosteroid doses (Kunz and Schreiner 1982, etc.). Prolonged treatment of rheumatic pregnant women with glucocorticoids can lead to adrenal cortex hypofunction in the fetus due to decreased production of ACTH; neonates in such cases reveal congenital adrenal insufficiency manifested in salt-losing crises and a drop in 17-ketosteroid (17-KS) and 17-oxyketosteroid (17-OKS) excretion (Kirushchenkov 1978). Long-term use of corticosteroids in the second and third trimesters can give rise to placental insifficiency (Stirrat 1976).

Salicylates, widely used in the therapy of rheumatic fever, had a teratogenic effect in experiments using relatively high drug doses (facial bones and skeleton anomalies). The dysmorphogenetic effect of salicylates in humans is not documented. Disturbances in erythrocyte metabolism, hyperbilirubinemia, nuclear jaundice, as well as delayed blood coagulation were noted in the newborn of mothers receiving high doses of acetylsalicylic acid near term (Pepperell 1983). In mothers salicylates also cause platelet dysfunction and delayed blood coagulation, which can become a serious threat during labor. Salicylates, especially in high doses, should not be given to pregnant women in the first 8 weeks of gestation (high salicylate doses are not recommended in pregnancy in general as there is a risk of placental separation). Retrospective epidemiological studies by Lewis and Schulman (1973) have shown that in women receiving 3.25 g acetylsalicylic acid/day in the third trimester of pregnancy, gestational and labor periods were prolonged, which is undesirable in cardiac patients. This can be attributed to prostaglandin synthetase inhibition. Other antiinflammatory agents, inhibiting prostaglandin synthetase (indomethacin, naproxen, etc.), used in antirheumatic therapy have the same effect (Kunz and Schreiner 1982; etc.). In addition, high doses of these drugs can cause premature closure of the ductus arteriosus in the fetus induced by the same mechanism (Kunz and Schreiner 1982). Indomethacin can also cause pulmonary hypertension in neonates (Pepperell 1983). All the above complications can be avoided with the drug withdrawal in the third trimester of pregnancy or at least several weeks before labor. Its use in the first and second trimesters of pregnancy is believed harmless for both the mother and fetus (except for cases of drug intolerance).

Cardiac glycosides, though quite easily crossing the placenta, possess neither teratogenic nor embryotoxic properties and can be used in their usual doses during pregnancy (Allonen et al. 1976; Rotmensch et al. 1983). This digoxin property can be used for transplacental relief of supraventricular tachycardia in the fetus (Kereni et al. 1980).

Anticoagulants, often used in patients at risk of thromboembolic complications (some forms of valvular heart disease, prosthetic cardiac valves, thrombophlebitis), must be used with utmost caution in pregnancy. Heparin, having a high molecular weight, cannot pass through the placenta and, therefore, has no effect on blood coagulation of the fetus and newborn. Indirect-acting anticoagulants (dicoumarol, warfarin, phenindione, etc.) easily pass through the placental barrier (irrespective of their almost complete binding to blood plasma proteins), delaying blood coagulation in the fetus (sometimes more than in the mother). Meningeal hemorrhage and hemorrhages in the inner organs can occur in the fetus. The embryotoxic action of coumarin derivatives is associated with the fact that the fetal liver is still incapable of producing detoxicating enzymes. Retroplacental hemorrhages are also possible, infrequently leading to fetal loss. The parallel use of indirect-acting anticoagulants and barbiturates, causing induction of hepatic microsomal enzymes in the mother (and therefore enhancing coumarin derivative metabolism) but having no similar effect on the fetus, constitute the greatest risk. The use of these anticoagulants near term can be the cause of life-threatening bleedings in the newborn (Stevenson et al. 1980).

Numerous cases have been reported of the teratogenic effect of indirect-acting anticoagulants used in the first trimester of pregnancy (Pettifor and Benson 1975; Kunz and Schreiner 1982). Fetal malformations are most frequent when coumarin derivatives are used in the 6th–9th week of pregnancy. Fetal malformations (including facial bones and skeleton anomalies, eye anomalies, up to optic nerve atrophy) (Iams and Rayborn 1982) and mental retardation of the child are often termed "warfarin embryopathy." The central nervous system may be damaged any time during pregnancy (Kunz and Schreiner 1982). The use of warfarin in late pregnancy can also cause hemorrhagic complications leading to fetal death (Lutz et al. 1978). However, Hirsch et al. (1972) gave warfarin to pregnant women for 14 weeks without any serious hemorrhagic complications in the fetus and the newborn. There have also been other singular reports on the absence of fetal complications with the use of coumarin derivatives (Hirsch et al. 1970; Stirrat 1976). Nevertheless, in two-thirds of 450 pregnancies when coumarin derivatives were used, the neonates were apparently normal; in one-third of the cases the infants had malformations or other complications, or pregnancy ended in spontaneous abortions and stillbirths (Hall et al. 1980). Certainly, this is too great a risk!

Adequate doses of indirect-acting anticoagulants usually cause no hemorrhagic complications in women during pregnancy, labor, and puerperium. But such complications have sometimes been observed with the use of heparin (Hall et al. 1980). In addition, constant use of heparin throughout the entire gestational period is probably associated with a certain risk of premature labor and stillbirth (Hall et al. 1980; Iams and Rayborn 1982). However, heparin is preferable in thromboembolic complications and for the prevention of these complications in pregnant women. In any case, in the first trimester of pregnancy anticoagulant therapy and prophylaxis should be performed only with heparin. If the woman in this period did receive coumarin preparations she should be warned of possible complications, and if the drug was used in the first 12 weeks of gestation termination of pregnancy should be considered.

Barbiturates, used for intravenous anesthesia, have no damaging effect on the fetus, though they pass freely through the placental barrier and accumulate in the fetal organs. But when the drugs are injected during labor shortly before birth, the newborn can develop respiratory insufficiency of varying degree due to suppression of the respiratory center function. Nitrous oxide and ether have the same effects on the respiratory center. If these two anesthetic agents are also used after induction of general anesthesia with barbiturates in cesarean section, the newborn can develop apnea. Therefore, in this case it is preferable to use propanidid, which has no depressing effect on the respiratory center of the fetus. Though Nelson and Forfar (1971) suggested that oral application of barbiturates as hypnotic drugs in early pregnancy can increase the incidence of congenital malformations, it is known that a great number of neonates born to mothers who attempted suicide with a large oral dose of barbiturates showed no malformations. However, the newborn of mothers who received high barbiturate doses throughout pregnancy and in the last trimester developed a so-called addiction syndrome on day 6–12 of the postnatal period that required the administration of phenobarbital or chlorpromazine (Tuchmann-Duplessis 1975). It is advisable to avoid the use of barbiturates in the first trimester of pregnancy, near term, or during labor.

Benzodiazepine compounds, nitrazepam, diazepam, chlordiazepoxide, oxazepam, and others, used in pregnancy as tranquilizers, pass easily through the placenta, having no detrimental effect on the fetus. Separate reports on the teratogenic effect of chlordiazepoxide and meprobamate (a tranquilizer from another group) used in early pregnancy were not confirmed in large prospective studies (Hartz et al. 1975; etc.). However, Mashkovsky (1984) does not recommend using tranquilizers in the first trimester of pregnancy.

Propranolol frequently used in patients with arterial hypertension and heart rhythm disturbances is inadvisable in pregnancy for long-term prevention (but not relief) of arrhythmias, though the views on this point are conflicting. It will suffice to note that in some cases long-term use of this drug by pregnant women caused intrauterine growth retardation as well as respiratory disorders (especially in cesarean section), bradycardia, hypoglycemia, and heart failure in newborns (Gladstone et al. 1975; Cottrill et al. 1977; Lighter et al. 1977). The syndrome of Q-T interval prolongation seems to be the only exclusion, as in this case propranolol is the most effective drug of choice (Wenger 1978). However, in recent years beta-blockers (sotalol, metoprolol, atenolol, etc.) have become more widerly used in pregnant women for the treatment of arterial hypertension, arrhythmias, and obstructive hypertrophic cardiomyopathy (idopathic hypertrophic subaortic stenosis).

Phenytoin (diphenylhydantoin) sometimes used as an antiarrhythmic agent freely passes through the placenta. When it is used in pregnancy, the incidence of fetal malformations (cardiac defects, cleft lip and palate), mental retardation, and other disturbances is higher than in the entire population (Iams and Rayborn 1982; Kunz and Schreiner 1982; etc.). With the use of phenytoin in the third trimester of pregnancy, fetal hemorrhages can be observed (Pepperell 1983; etc.). All the disorders were observed with the drug used as an antiepileptic agent. But, since the teratogenic effect of the drug cannot be disputed, it is contraindicated in early pregnancy. Short-term phenytoin application in the second and third trimesters of pregnancy for relief of paroxysmal arrhythmias (especially in digitalis intoxication and refractoriness to lidocaine and beta-blockers) might be possible.

Antiarrhythmic drugs, containing ajmalin — an alkaloid of *Rauwolfia* — may cause rhinitis in the newborn and, therefore, should be withdrawn 1–2 weeks before labor (Kunz and Schreiner 1982).

Quinidine used for antiarrhythmic therapy should be avoided in the first trimester of gestation; later in pregnancy high drug doses cannot be used either. Though there is an opinion that quinidine might cause premature labor (Bellet 1972), it was established that the oxytocic effect of quinidine is minimal and starts only with spontaneous uterine contractions (Szekely and Snaith 1974). Lidocaine as an antiarrhythmic agent should not be used in very high doses. Though it (like procainamide used for the same purpose) does not have a teratogenic effect, its toxic doses in fetal acidosis can cause depression of the central nervous and cardiovascular systems in the fetus.

Though it is believed that amiodarone may have an adverse effect on the fetus due to the high iodine content in it (Kunz and Schreiner 1982), there are reports on the absence of side effects during its administration in pregnancy (McKenna et al. 1983; Pitcher et al. 1983; Robson et al. 1985; Penn et al. 1985).

The drugs used in hyperthyroidism (propylthiouracil, iodine-containing preparations, including radioactive iodine) freely pass through the placenta, depressing the function of the fetal thyroid gland. This stimulates thyrotrophic hormone secretion, causes hypertrophy of the fetal thyroid gland, and the neonate has goiter. In some cases, the enlarged thyroid gland of the fetus can obstruct the trachea, possibly causing death due to suffocation (Tuchmann-Duplessis 1975). Suppression of thyroxine synthesis by the fetal thyroid gland may be the cause of congenital hypothyroidism and functional insufficiency of the central nervous system.

10.3.2 Management of Patients with Rheumatic Heart Disease

Pregnancy is not a contraindication for regular secondary preventive therapy with penicillin. With rheumatic fever exacerbation, the patient should be hospitalized; bed rest, reduced salt and carbohydrate diet, and increased consumption of animal proteins, vegetables, and fruit are indicated. Additional vitamin intake is advisable. Because of their effect on the fetus, glucocorticoids should be used only in a rheumatic process of high activity and beginning not earlier than in the second trimester of pregnancy and for not very long periods. Daily doses of prednisolone (and prednisone), dexamethasone, and triamcinolone are 10–20 mg, 2–3 mg, and 8–16 mg, respectively. The latter drug has the least, as compared with the above drugs, effect on the sodium and water balance, and, therefore, it may be used in patients with heart failure. In rheumatic fever, first degree of activity, acetylsalicylic acid at a daily dose of 4–6 g or aminophenazole at a dose of 2–2.5 g may prove effective. As phenylbutazone has a negative effect on the water-electrolyte balance, leukopoiesis, and blood coagulation, it should be avoided in pregnancy. In rheumatic fever, second and third degree of activity, combined therapy with glucocorticoids and nonsteroid antiinflammatory agents is performed. The therapy is continued until the signs of the rheumatic process disappear (usually for 1–1.5 months). In severe rheumatic carditis and manifestations of heart failure strict bed rest is indicated (lying supine in bed can reduce the cardiac preload due to partial obstruction of the inferior vena cava by the enlarged uterus); water and salt consumption should be limited to 600 to 800 ml/day and 3 g/day, respectively. Along with antirheumatic agents, cardiac glycosides (preferably with minimal cumulative effect) and, if necessary, diuretics (hydrochlorothiazide, furosemide) are indicated. In some cases diuretics should be given before the treatment with glycosides is started. To prevent hypokalemia, administration of potassium salts is required. At early stages of heart failure digoxin is administered orally (with the beginning of the labor period glycosides are administered intravenously): on the first day — 0.25 mg four times daily (loading dose), on the following days — 0.25 mg one to three times daily. Administration of usual digitoxin doses is possible. However, its clearance is slow, and as the hemodynamic situation in pregnancy can rapidly change, sometimes requiring intravenous cardiac glycoside injections or cardioversion, digoxin seems preferable. In pregnant women with severe heart failure, when orally administered drugs are poorly absorbed (due to "congestive stomach") cardiac glycosides should be injected intravenously. Daily control over heart rate and diuresis, as well as regular (e.g., every 5 days) ECG recordings, are obligatory to adjust effective individual doses of glycosides and avoid glycoside intoxication (loss of appetite, nausea, vomiting, bradycardia, bigeminy, premature beats, AV block), requiring immediate discontinuation of glycoside therapy. It should be noted that pregnant women are sometimes administered high doses of calcium chloride for obstetric indications, which constitutes a significant threat during treatment with cardiac glycosides and may be a cause of death from ventricular fibrillation. Vasodilators play an important role in the treatment of heart failure. Nitrates (sublingual nitroglycerin, isosorbide dinitrate — oral dose 20–60 mg six times a day), causing venous dilation, reduce pulmonary congestion. Hydralazine (25–100 mg three to four times a day), which has a vasodilating effect on arterioles, contributes to the decrease in peripheral vascular resistance and thus to cardiac output increase. Prazosin affects both the venous system and arterioles; its initial oral dose should not exceed 1 mg. However, during pregnancy, these drugs are probably to be used only in acute cases, as their long-term use may have an adverse effect on the fetus by reducing uterine-placental blood flow. In acute cases (pulmonary edema) controlled use of sodium nitroprusside is possible in the absence of hypotension. Its initial infusion rate is 10 μg/min, it is increased by 5–10 μg/min every 5 min until the pulmonary edema is relieved or hypotension is achieved.

Diuretic doses are individually adjusted: hydrochlorothiazide, from 25 to 100 mg per day; furosemide, 40–120 mg/day. Depending on the severity of edema, diuretics are given daily, every other day or one to two times a week. Spironolactone (100 to 200 mg/day) and triamterene (50–150 mg/day) are used. The drugs have no marked diuretic effect, but reduce the potassium loss caused by other diuretics. Spironolactone should not be given in the first trimester of pregnancy. In thromboembolic complications diuretics should be used with caution. In streptococcal infection penicillin therapy (at a dose not less than 1200000 units/day) is performed. In patients with heart disease, when there is a risk of bacterial endocarditis, therapy with antibiotics should be performed before and after labor.

The treatment of cardiac asthma and pulmonary edema during pregnancy is conventional, but it must be intensive and urgent. To reduce venous return the patient should be placed in the "trunk up — legs down" position, and the tourniquets can be applied to her extremities. It is advisable to apply the cuffs to the proximal thigh or shoulder areas and pump them 10 mmHg below diastolic BP level. This does not prevent arterial flow, considerably limiting venous return (Ingram and Braunwald 1984). Tourniquets can be applied simultaneously to two or three extremities, with one tourniquet moved to the free extremity every 15 min. They are gradually removed. In the presence of thrombophlebitis or leg edema tourniquets are not applied on the legs. Blood-letting is inadvisable in pregnant women, and 0.5–0.75 ml 0.05% ouabaine (strophanthine G) or 1 ml 0.025% digoxin (previous digitalization should be taken into consideration; glycosides should not be injected intravenously if 24 h have not passed since the last oral digoxin dose) and 40–60 mg furosemide are slowly infused intravenously. If cardiac glycosides are undesirable for fear of glycoside intoxication, the furosemide dose can be increased to 120–240 mg. Slow intravenous injections of 1 ml thalamonal (or 1 ml 0.25% droperidol and 1 ml 0.005% fentanyl) are possible. However, it would be better not to use the latter drug during labor and especially in cesarean section, as it depresses fetal respiration and in high doses may suppress uterine contractions. If pulmonary edema develops in the puerperium, thalamonal (droperidol and fentanyl) may be safely used.

During treatment of pulmonary edema, 0.5 ml atropine can be injected subcutaneously (promethazine hydrochloride or diphenhydramine chloride can be used instead of atropine). It should be taken into consideration that morphine commonly used for the reduction of respiratory center excitability also depresses fetal respiration and, therefore, its use immediately before and during labor should be avoided.

Patients with cardiac asthma are treated by inhalation of oxygen-enriched gas at a rate of 4–6 liters/min.

With the onset of heart failure symptoms associated with rheumatic fever recurrence in the first trimester of gestation, pregnancy should be terminated, as the prognosis is poor.

10.3.3 Management of Patients with Congenital Heart Disease

The management of pregnant women with congenital heart disease is conventional. Prevention of heart failure is essential and with the onset of the first symptoms the management is the same as in rheumatic valvular heart disease. Heart failure increases the risk of thromboembolic complications especially in some congenital heart diseases (see Chap. 5); therefore, preventive therapy with heparin is advisable in severe heart failure.

Though it is preferable to correct surgically curable cardiac lesions prior to pregnancy or some time after delivery, in some cases cardiosurgeons have to operate on pregnant patients threatened with sudden and prompt onset of heart failure. Mostly, these are patients with mitral stenosis in whom valvotomy abolishes hemodynamic disturbances and decreases cardiac load. Perioperative mortality of patients operated on in due time during pregnancy does not at present exceed their perioperative mortality in the prepregnant period. It should be noted that in acquired heart disease surgical intervention is possible only in the absence of an active rheumatic process. Before surgery it seems necessary to remove manifestations of heart failure, which, nowadays, with the development of new inotropic drugs and wide use of vasodilators, has become an easier task than when the physicians had to make do only with cardiac glycosides and not always potent diuretics. However, new and old drugs as well should be used with caution. For instance, excessive use of diuretics and limited liquid consumption in patients with aortic stenosis can dramatically reduce an already insufficient preload. Vasodilators in these patients can lower an already decreased coronary perfusion and beta-blockers and calcium antagonists in severe stenosis may render the patient incapable of increasing cardiac output in response to physical exercise. Sufficient preload should be maintained in patients with Eisenmenger's syndrome and primary pulmonary hypertension (care should be taken not to abuse diuretics, if indicated, and excessive use of vasodilators should be avoided).

10.3.4 Cardiosurgery During Pregnancy

Though the operation of choice in mitral stenosis is closed valvotomy, nowadays annuloplasty and valve replacement are sometimes performed. Biological prostheses, requiring no anticoagulant therapy, are preferable (porcine or human cadaver tissue valves). If not biological, artificial mostly cloth-covered prosthetic valves are implanted. Bearing in mind the high incidence of complications during implantation of rigid prosthetic valves to pregnant women, valvotomy seems preferable in this period. It should also be recognized that open heart surgery early in pregnancy is associated with great teratogenic risk. Surgery is preferable in the 18th–24th week of gestation. However, in life-threatening conditions (refractory pulmonary edema, massive hemoptysis) mitral valvotomy can be performed at any time during pregnancy. In pregnancy, surgical treatment can be performed, if indicated, in aortic stenosis, coarctation of the aorta, congenital heart disease, and subacute bacterial endocarditis. Long-term antirheumatic therapy in rheumatic valvular heart disease is performed after surgery. Pregnant women with nonbiological prosthetic cardiac valves should be subcutaneously administered 20000–25000 units of heparin/day to avoid the teratogenic effect of coumarin anticoagulants in the first trimester of pregnancy and to avoid hemorrhagic complications caused by the latter in the third trimester of pregnancy. Thrombin time should exceed normal about 2–2.5-fold (Deeg 1983). There are proponents of heparin use only in the first 12 and last 4 weeks of gestation, with the application of more effective warfarin in the remaining periods (Murnaghan 1982). During therapy Quick's index should be 10%–15%. An attempt to use low-heparin doses (500 units every 12 h) at the same periods in women with prosthetic cardiac valves did not provide adequate thromboembolic prophylaxis (Wang et al. 1983). Preventive use of antithrombotic drug combinations (acetylsalicylic acid, pentoxifylline, dipyridamole) with each other and with warfarin were attempted in patients with prosthetic cardiac valves (Chesebro 1983; Mok et al. 1985). The attempts to replace warfarin by antithrombotic drugs (or merely reduce its doses) were futile, though Biale et al. (1980) reported on the successful use of dipyridamole, acetylsalicylic acid, and warfarin combination.

10.3.5 Management of Patients with Nonrheumatic Myocarditis

Irrespective of the etiology of the disease in pregnant women, bed rest and sodium and water restriction are indicated. The choice of the way of management depends on the etiology and severity of myocarditis. Specific treatment is performed in fungal myocarditis, while in bacterial, viral, ricketsial, and parasitary myocarditis it is necessary to treat the underlying disease. In severe or protracted myocarditis the same antiinflammatory drugs as in rheumatic fever are given. In torpid or recurring myocarditis (including rheumatic carditis) the treatment with quinoline derivatives (0.2–0.5 g chloroquine/day) can be started immediately after labor and can last for 6–9 months. In myocarditis that has allergic manifestations, moderate doses of corticosteroids are used for a short period during pregnancy, with the doses increased to the usual level after delivery. Antihistamine agents are less effective and should be used only when glucocorticoids are contraindicated (e.g., in viral myocarditis). Antibradykinin agents seem expedient (namely, 0.75–1.0 g pyridinolcarbamate/day).

Anabolic steroids should be avoided during pregnancy because of their possible effect on the fetus. In cases complicated by heart failure, cardiac glycosides and diuretics in combination with potassium preparations are used. In marked cardialgia analgesics are given; the feeling of discomfort in the chest occasionally disappears with the use of mild sedative drugs (valerian and so forth). Infrequent monofocal premature beats require no special treatment. In other heart rhythm disturbances, if arrhythmia persists after treatment with antiinflammatory drugs, antiarrhythmic therapy is indicated. The treatment of myocarditis should be long-term even in the absence of a recurrent inflammatory process.

10.3.6 Management of Patients with Hypertrophic Cardiomiopathy

The treatment of patients with hypertrophic cardiomyopathy is, as a rule, symptomatic. Long-term application of beta-blockers conventionally used for the treatment of angina and arrhythmias is inadvisable in pregnancy, as cases of placental immaturity, fetal bradycardia, and low birth weight of neonates following such therapy have been reported. However, Rubin et al. (1983) have noted only bradycardia in infants born to mothers with hypertrophic cardiomyopathy receiving atenolol. Beta-blockers are contraindicated in patients with heart failure. The feasibility of using calcium channel blockers in pregnant women with hypertrophic cardiomyopathy has not been studied so far. As there is a risk of bacterial endocarditis, preventive therapy with antibiotics seems expedient in the ante- and postpartal periods. The operation of partial excision of the hypertrophic myocardium should not be performed in pregnancy.

10.3.7 Management of Patients with Peripartal Cardiomyopathy

There is no specific treatment of the disease. Urgent hospitalization, strict bed rest, and sodium restriction are required. If the disease developed before labor, the patient should assume the supine position, promoting preload reduction. Heart failure is treated as in valvular heart disease. Digitalization should be performed with utmost caution, as there is an increased risk of digitalis intoxication in patients with peripartal cardiomyopathy, infrequently mediated by hypokalemia and hypomagnesemia. In acute heart failure, controlled use of vasodilators is possible. When peripartal cardiomyopathy is believed to be the result of preceding myocarditis, immunodepressive therapy with corticosteroids and azathioprine should be performed. Azathioprine, though devoid of teratogenic effect in humans, has an adverse effect on the fetus (Kunz and Schreiner 1982; etc.), and, therefore, it should be used with caution. In the presence of thromboembolic complications or arrhythmias an appropriate therapy should be performed. Preventive therapy of thromboembolism with heparin seems expedient during pregnancy; and in the puerperium the use of coumarin anticoagulants is possible.

10.3.8 Management of Patients with Thyrotoxic Heart Muscle Disease

The treatment is mainly symptomatic. Iodine drugs and thiamazol, as well as propylthiouracil, pose a threat to the fetus. Surgery on the maternal thyroid gland is the safest procedure for the fetus. The best time for surgery is the beginning of the second trimester of pregnancy. Short-term use of 0.015–0.02 g thiamozol/day in the preoperative period is possible; however, it may increase blood loss during the operation; therefore, the drug should be withdrawn 1–2 weeks before surgery. In the third stage of labor and the early puerperium hemorrhages due to alterations in the blood coagulation system can arise.

10.3.9 Management of Patients with Anemic Heart Muscle Disease

The treatement of patients with anemia depends on the underlying cause. Preventive therapy to remove anemia is obligatory (even in the absence of symptoms of heart muscle disease) if the hemoglobin level is below 100–110 g/liter (at this level anemia is always genuine, but not dilutional). In the case of iron-deficiency anemia, iron-containing drugs are administered orally. High doses of ascorbic acid are indicated. In intolerance to oral iron-containing drugs they are injected intramuscularly or intravenously. In B_{12} — and folic-deficiency anemia 100–200 μg vitamin B_{12} is injected intramuscularly and 4–5 mg/day folic acid is administered orally every day.

10.3.10 Management of Patients with Myocardial Infarction

For urgent pain relief 10 mg morphine (with 0.5 mg atropine) or 4 mg dihydromorphinone is subcutaneously or intravenously injected slowly. If the woman is not in labor, thalamonal or a mixture containing 1–2 ml 0.25% droperidol and 1–2 ml 0.005% fentanyl in 20 ml 40% glucose is slowly infused intravenously. If possible, anesthesia is performed with a nitrous oxide-oxygen mixture (the initial ratio is 80 to 20, and then the nitrous oxide concentration is reduced to 50% with the oxygen concentration increased accordingly). Anticoagulant therapy is carried out; 10000 to 15000 units heparin (preferably intravenously) comprise the initial dose, then every 4–6 h 5000–10000 units is injected with daily control over the clotting and partial thromboplastin time (it should be 1.5–2.5 times higher than normal). The treatment lasts for 1–2 weeks. With patients intolerant to heparin, indirect-acting anticoagulants are used. In this case, the prothrombin index (which should be 40%–50%) is to be controlled. In the case of roentgenologically verified coronary artery thrombosis streptokinase can also be used for thrombolysis: 1000000 units of the drug for 1/2 h or 1500000 units for 1 h is intravenously infused. Then heparin therapy is started. Streptodekase synthesized in the Soviet Union is a preparation that retains potent concentration and high fibrinolytic activity for 48–72 h after a single injection. Its therapeutic dose is 3000000 units (the contents of two to three vials). The drug (each vial) is diluted in 10–20 ml sterile apyrogenic isotonic sodium chloride solution. Initially, a bolus streptodekase dose (300000 units) is intravenously injected for the neutralization of possible streptococcal antigens and the assessment of individual drug tolerance. If the drug is well tolerated, 1 h after the first intravenous injection the remaining 2700000 units of streptodekase is administered intravenously for 3–5 min. Twenty-four hours later heparin therapy can be started (usually 40000 units per day) with consideration of the clotting time. Streptodekase injection can be repeated no sooner than 3–6 months later. The drugs (streptokinase and streptodekase) are not recommended in the first 18 weeks of pregnancy and the first 4 days of the puerperium. Care should be taken as to the use of thrombolytic agents during pregnancy, as they may cause bleedings, allergic conditions, and pyrogenic reactions. In the case of bleeding 100 ml 5% aminocaproic acid is intravenously infused (it is important to bear in mind that the drug passes through the placenta and, therefore, protamine sulfate is preferable in heparin-induced bleedings); if need be, the drip infusions can be repeated at 4-h intervals. In allergic conditions or pyrogenic reactions, diphenhydramine chloride or chloropyramine is intravenously injected. The same drugs are intravenously injected before streptokinase administration for the prevention of pyrogenic reactions.

Prevention of arrhythmias is ensured by intravenous administration of a 1% lidocaine solution within 2 days after onset of the disease: first 100-mg bolus injection and then drip infusion at a rate of 1–3 mg/min. The same drug is used for the treatment of arrhythmias; a 100- to 150-mg bolus injection is followed by drip infusion at a rate of 1–4 mg/min. When ventricular premature beats compromise hemodynamics slow intravenous injections of procainamide can be used (the initial dose is 2.5 ml of a 10% solution, then 1 ml of the drug is injected repeatedly at 5-min intervals; the total dose should not exceed 1000 mg). If procainamide infusion is fast BP may fall. Procainamide may also be given orally (first — 0.75–1 g, then 0.25–0.5 g every 3–4 h). In rare cases (and only after the 12th week of pregnancy) may more toxic drugs — quinidine sulfate and quinidine bisulfate — be used (to exclude possible allergic reactions, the initial oral dose 0.1–0.2 g is given, followed by 0.2–0.3 g of the drug every 4–6 h). Ajmalin (gilurytmal) (50 mg intravenously or intramuscularly three to four times a day), verapamil (5–10 mg intravenously and then 40 mg orally every 4 h), and cardiac glycosides are applied for the treatment of arrhythmias. Propranolol and diphenylhydantoin should not be used in pregnancy; however, if they are indispensable and apparently effective, their short-term use seems possible. In sinus bradycardia and atrioventricular and sinoatrial block, subcutaneous or intravenous injection of 0.5–1 mg atropine can sometimes prove very effective. Repeated atropine injections should be avoided, as this drug relaxes the cervical muscles. In atrial fibrillation refractory to medical therapy DC countershock is performed. Temporary electrical heart stimulation may be performed in brady- and tachyarrhythmias or heart blocks.

10.3.11 Management of Patients with Subacute Bacterial Endocarditis

Large doses of antibiotics are administered. The drug dose depends on the agent's sensitivity. Before the results of blood culture are obtained, treatment with penicillin is started at 3- or 4-h intervals, with a daily dose of 6000000–12000000 units. Penicillin therapy lasts for 1–1.5 months and is combined in the first 2 weeks with 0.5 g streptomycin every 12 h. If *Staphylococcus* revealed in the culture does not produce penicillinase, the daily penicillin dose can be increased to 25000000–50000000 units, which permits shortening the treatment period to 1 month. If the *Staphylococcus* does produce penicillinase, methicillin (2–4 g every 4 h), oxacillin (1–2 g every 4 h), or lincomycin (only if other drugs prove ineffective, 0.5 g every 8 h) are administered intramuscularly. Kanamycin, vancomycin, and gentamicin should be avoided in pregnancy. Cephalosporin antibiotics can be used only commencing with the second trimester of pregnancy. When the pathogenic flora is refractory to antibiotics, the patients are administered antistaphylococcal plasma or γ-globulin. In the case of *Staphylococcus viridans* cephaloridine (cephalexin) (0.5 g every 6 h) is injected intramuscularly but only beginning with the second trimester of pregnancy. If *Enterococcus* is revealed in the culture, 20000000–40000000 units/day of penicillin and 1 g/day of streptomycin are given. Ampicillin, which in endocarditis is usually applied in high doses, is not used in pregnancy. Endocarditis can be prevented by the treatment of any infection occurring in pregnancy, elimination of infective foci, and prophylactic use of antibiotics during minor interventions (catheterization, dental extraction, etc.). It is especially true for pregnant women with diseases predisposing to the development of endocarditis.

10.3.12 Management of Patients with Pericarditis

The patients with acute pericarditis require bed rest. The underlying disease (if known) should be treated and acetylsalicylic acid is administered. In idiopathic pericarditis corticosteroids are effective. In threatened heart tamponade pericardial puncture is performed using the subxiphoidal or other approach and pericardial exudate is slowly aspirated. To avoid severe heart failure in patients with constrictive pericarditis, pericardectomy, if necessary, is performed during pregnancy.

10.3.13 Management of Patients with Heart Rhythm Disturbances

In arrhythmias the drug choice is often determined not only by the type of cardiac rhythm disorder, but also by the individual drug sensitivity. Before the treatment is started, Holter ECG monitoring should be performed in pregnant women with arrhythmias, including heart blocks, to specify the type of rhythm and conduction disturbances. First of all, arrhythmogenic factors should be removed (smoking, strong tea or coffee abuse, thyrotoxicosis, myocarditis, glycoside intoxication, etc.). Sometimes heart rhythm disturbances in pregnant women respond to valerian and other sedatives or tranquilizers.

10.3.13.1 Atrial and Atrioventricular Nodal Premature Beats

These premature beats do not commonly require any special treatment. However, frequent and coupled supraventricular premature beats may foretell the onset of atrial fibrillation in pregnant women with mitral stenosis, and, therefore, require preventive use of verapamil (20–40 mg two to three times/day) or ajmalin (50–100 mg three times/day); the latter drug must be withdrawn 1–2 weeks before term. To control premature beats 10 ml 10% potassium chloride can also be given orally three to four times/day. If premature beat results from untreated heart failure they can disappear with the use of cardiac glycosides (it should be remembered that premature beats can also be caused by glycoside intoxication; in this case they disappear with glycoside discontinuation). Occasionally, procainamide (0.25–0.5 g every 3–4 h) or quinidine (0.1–0.2 g every 6–8 h) can prove effective; the latter drug is used only beginning with the 13th week of pregnancy. Administration of minor tranquilizers or beta-blockers can also be successful (Rotmensch et al. 1983).

10.3.13.2 Ventricular Premature Beats

Infrequent and late ventricular premature beats do not require treatment if they are tolerated fairly well. If necessary, the treatment is the same as in atrial premature beats. Intensive therapy of frequent, early, polyfocal, and coupled ventricular premature beats threatening with ventricular tachycardia and fibrillation is obligatory. If premature beats in pregnant women are secondary to sinus bradycardia, the injection of 0.5–1 ml of 0.1% atropine or oral administration of belladonna (tincture or powder) may be effective. In other cases, lidocaine (intravenously), procainamide, verapamil, ajmalin, and potassium preparations are given orally; short-term use of propafenon (300–600 mg/day) is possible. If ventricular (and supraventricular) premature beats are manifestations of digitalis intoxication or hypersensitivity to glycosides in patients with heart failure, cardiac glycosides and diuretics should be discontinued for 3–5 days, with glycoside therapy (if indispensable) resumed later in lower doses. In digitalis intoxication short-term administration of phenytoin is possible in the second and third trimesters of pregnancy.

10.3.13.3 Sinus Tachycardia

Sinus tachycardia, being usually a symptom of some disease, can be eliminated by adequate therapy of the underlying disease. Ajmalin (50–100 mg three times, daily), digoxin (12.5–25 mg/day), and tranquilizers are given, and short-term application of verapamil (40–80 mg three times daily) is possible.

10.3.13.4 Paroxysmal Tachycardia

Therapy is started after urgent ECG recording, as the treatment in supraventricular and ventricular forms is different. Short paroxysms of supraventricular tachycardia are usually well tolerated, and can, therefore, go untreated.

Supraventricular paroxysmal tachycardia (atrial and atrioventricular nodal reentrant) is sometimes eliminated with sedatives and minor tranquilizers. Vagus stimulation by unilateral massage of the carotid sinus, pressure on the eyeballs, Valsalva's maneuver, and gagging may sometimes be effective. The attack can be arrested by slow intravenous injection of 2–4 ml 0.25% verapamil, 3–5 ml 0.01% propranolol, 0.25–0.5 ml 0.05% ouabain, 1 ml 0.025% digoxin, or 5–10 ml 10% procainamide. If the attack is accompanied by a drop in BP, 0.5–1 ml 1% phenylephrine is injected subcutaneously or intramuscularly. On rare occasions, when medical therapy is ineffective, cardioversion (it should not be used in digitalis intoxication) or electrical atrial or ventricular pacing are performed. In frequent attacks of tachycardia in pregnant women, preventive therapy with the usual doses of digoxin or digitoxin, ajmalin bitartrate (10–20 mg two to three times daily), procainamide (250–500 mg three times daily), or, if they are ineffective, amiodaron (200 mg two to three times daily) or propafenon (300–600 mg/day) are administered.

In ventricular paroxysmal tachycardia, mechanical vagus stimulation is of no use. Cardiac glycosides in this case are not recommended either. Urgent therapy should be started with intravenous lidocaine infusion (2.5–5 ml of a 2% solution should be first given as a bolus injection at a rate of about 20–50 mg/min and then dripped for 15–20 min, the total dose not exceeding 4–5 mg/kg) or slow intravenous injection of 5–10 ml 10% procainamide. Sometimes cardioversion is performed (in some cases the procedure is repeated). In mild cases single oral procainamide administration (0.75–1.5 g) followed by 0.25–0.5 g every 3 h may prove effective. If ventricular tachycardia does not respond to medical therapy, electrical cardioversion is employed. For the prevention of attacks, potassium salts, procainamide, verapamil, and lidocaine (in the presence of ventricular premature beats) are given orally and, if they prove ineffective, amiodarone, propafenon, and disopyramide (100–200 mg four times daily) are used.

10.3.13.5 Atrial Tachyarrhythmias

The management depends on the nature of arrhythmia (paroxysmal or stable) and its form (atrial flutter or fibrillation).

In *paroxysms of atrial fibrillation* 5–10 ml of a 10% procainamide solution is slowly injected intravenously. Sometimes 2 ml 0.1% propranolol or 2–4 ml 0.25% verapamil may prove effective. In patients with heart failure atrial fibrillation can be relieved by 0.5–0.75 ml 0.05% ouabain or 1 ml 0.025% digoxin; if there is no effect, 0.5 ml ouabain can be injected repeatedly 45–60 min later. Cardioversion is performed only in life-threatening conditions, though some authors (Schroeder and Harrison 1971) believe it necessary for the prevention of pulmonary edema in patients with mitral stenosis when coexisting arrhythmias are refractory to cardiac glycosides. In these cases, ouabain and digoxin should be discontinued 1–2 days before the procedure if there are no signs of glycoside intoxication.

In *atrial flutter*, contrastingly, direct-current cardioversion is the main method of treatment, as medical therapy is ineffective in the majority of cases. If a cardioverter is not available, the drugs of choice are verapamil, cardiac glycosides, and propranolol injected intravenously.

To prevent *atrial fibrillation* the usual doses of procainamide, verapamil, ajmalin bitartrate, and metoprolol are used; when they are ineffective, amiodarone (200 mg two to three times daily) or disopyramide (200 mg two to three times daily) are given.

In *persistent atrial fibrillation* of a relatively short duration (not more than 1 year), in the absence of considerable myocardial alterations, active myocarditis, pronounced atrial enlargement, severe heart failure, and serious conduction disturbances, an attempt can be made to recover sinus rhythm, considerably improve hemodynamic conditions in advancing pregnancy, and, to a certain extent, reduce the risk of thromboembolic complications. If the pregnant woman has mitral stenosis, it seems advisable, first of all, to correct it surgically (in appropriate indications and conditions). In heart failure cardiac glycosides and diuretics are given.

Two weeks before electrical cardioversion, therapy with indirect-acting anticoagulants is performed for the prevention of thromboembolic complications (the prothrombin index is to be maintained at a 50%–60% level). One to two days before cardioversion digoxin must be withdrawn, while cardiac glycosides whose elimination time is longer should be discontinued 3–4 days before the procedure. Electrical cardioversion is not performed in glycoside intoxication. As sinus rhythm restoration with high quinidine doses is contraindicated during pregnancy and procainamide is not sufficiently effective, direct-current cardioversion seems the only reliable method of treatment. After successful cardioversion, the pregnant woman should be kept on bed rest for 1–2 weeks and should continue receiving anticoagulants. Cardioversion should be performed under monitoring of fetal cardiac rhythm, though the energy of the discharge reaching the fetus is extremely low.

When stable recent atrial fibrillation is refractory to therapy, or if atrial fibrillation is long standing, the hemodynamic situation can, to a certain extent, be improved by decreasing the accelerated ventricular rate to 60–80/min or the reduction or complete relief of pulse deficit. Cardiac glycosides are used for this purpose. In severe cases, treatment can be started with intravenous injections (sometimes twice daily) of 0.5–0.75 ml 0.05% ouabain or 1 ml 0.025% digoxin followed by maintenance therapy with digoxin or other oral digitalis preparations. In less severe cases, a 1- to 2-day prompt loading with digoxin at a dose of 1–1.25 mg/day is performed, with the following maintenance doses of 0.125–0.5 mg/day adjusted according to the heart rate. Sensitivity to cardiac glycosides is variable; therefore, maintenance doses should be individually regulated. In pregnant women with chronic atrial fibrillation and thromboembolism in history, preventive use of heparin or indirect-acting anticoagulants seems advisable.

10.3.13.6 Wolff-Parkinson-White Syndrome

The Wolff-Parkinson-White (WPW) syndrome without tachyarrhythmia attacks requires no treatment. In pregnancy it is only necessary to reduce physical activity and exclude strong tea, coffee, and alcohol consumption, which might provoke attacks of supraventricular tachycardia. The treatment of supraventricular tachycardia paroxysms is conventional. In paroxysms of atrial flutter, or fibrillation secondary to the WPW syndrome, cardiac glycosides can not only be ineffective but also dangerous, and, therefore, it is better to avoid their use in such cases. The attack may be arrested by intravenous infusion of procainamide, verapamil, or propranolol, but the main way to eliminate atrial flutter or fibrillation is cardioversion. Digoxin, procainamide, propranolol, amiodarone (Penn et al. 1985), and long-acting quinidine are used for the prevention of arrhythmias. When medical therapy is ineffective, implantation of a pacemaker for the prevention of arrhythmias seems advisable. It can be performed during pregnancy. Surgical ablation of accessory atrioventricular pathways (and sometimes normal AV conduction tract) should be avoided during pregnancy.

10.3.13.7 Sinoatrial Block

Sinoatrial block with rare pauses requires no treatment. If the block is caused by cardiac glycoside overdose, the drugs should be discontinued. In other cases the block might be eliminated by oral atropine sulfate (0.5 mg four times daily) or intravenous injection of 0.5–1 mg atropine. In more severe cases, when bradycardia or bradycardia alternating with tachycardia attacks are poorly tolerated or when the block is accompanied by syncope (even seldom) pacemaker implantation is indicated as medical therapy in the majority of cases proves ineffective.

10.3.13.8 Atrioventricular Block

In AV block medical treatment is a bit more effective than in sinoatrial block; however, unfortunately, the effect is often short term. Women with congenital complete heart block and a ventricular rate of at least 50/min usually tolerate pregnancy fairly well and require no treatment. When the block is caused by cardiac glycosides the drugs are immediately discontinued. The degree of the block can be reduced by atropine injection, sublingual administration of 10–20 mg isoproterenol (isoprenaline), or injections of orciprenaline (0.5–1 ml of a 0.05% solution slowly intravenously or 1–2 ml intramuscularly or subcutaneously, or oral administration of 0.02 g of the drug every 3–4 h). It should be recognized that isoproterenol and orciprenaline can sometimes induce premature beats and even ventricular tachycardia, and suppress uterine contractions during labor. A more durable relief of complete heart block is achieved by prednisolone (20–30 mg/day) when the block is secondary to myocarditis. Short-term use of high drug doses (up to 120 mg/day) is possible in blocks secondary to myocardial infarction. In high-degree blocks, secondary to myocardial infarction, repeated intravenous injections of 0.5 mg atropine (total dose, 2 mg) at 1- to 2-min intervals may prove effective. AV block is most effectively treated by electrical ventricular stimulation (temporary pacemaker insertion — in transient block and permanent pacemaker insertion — in stable block). Temporary electrical heart stimulation is performed under local anesthesia using a transvenous pacing catheter most often inserted through the left subclavian vein and fixed in the endocardium. In case of emergency, transthoracic temporary electrical heart stimulation can be performed.

In *fascicular blocks* medical therapy is usually ineffective. When there is a complete intraventricular block pacemaker implantation is necessary.

In *Adams-Stokes attacks* emergency aid is necessary: closed-chest cardiac massage and injections of 0.02% isoproterenol (1–2 ml to 5 ml, subcutaneously or intramuscularly, or 1 ml intravenously). Intravenous drip infusions of 5–15 mg isoproterenol or 2.5–7.5 mg orciprenaline in 500 ml of a 5% glucose solution or physiological saline seem expedient in hospital conditions under ECG control and constant BP measurements. Subcutaneous or intramuscular injections of 0.5–1 ml 0.1% atropine, 0.5 ml 0.1% epinephrine, or 1 ml 5% ephedrine may prove effective. In cases refractory to medical therapy, temporary electrical heart stimulation is performed with following pacemaker implantation.

10.3.14 Preventive Treatment of Patients with Prosthetic Cardiac Valves

In pregnant women with prosthetic cardiac valves heparin should be substituted for indirect-acting anticoagulants at the very beginning of the gestational period. In the second trimester of pregnancy it is preferable to continue heparin. In the third trimester indirect-acting anticoagulants are possible, but they should again be replaced by heparin 2 weeks before term. Though some authors (Deeg 1983; etc.) believe the use of coumarin derivatives by breast-feeding mothers inadvisable, the amount of anticoagulants penetrating maternal milk seems negligible. And thus, gradual transition to indirect-acting anticoagulants after delivery is possible.

11 Labor and Termination of Pregnancy in Women with Cardiovascular Diseases

Pregnant women with cardiovascular diseases are admitted to a special high-risk pregnancy unit of a maternity hospital 3–4 weeks before delivery to prepare them for childbirth by treating heart failure, heart rhythm disturbances, and arterial hypertension or when necessary to discontinue the drugs that are undesirable immediately before and during labor. It is also advisable to hospitalize the patients with cardiovascular diseases in advance as they usually have labor 1–3 weeks before term (Kofler et al. 1982).

11.1 Management of Labor in Patients with Cardiovascular Diseases

Delivery at term by cesarean section was earlier believed to reduce cardiac load and to decrease mortality rate among pregnant women with heart diseases. Now cesarean section in such patients is recommended only when obstetrically indicated. However, some authors (Avar et al. 1976; Taurelle and Duhon 1976) do advise delivery by cesarean section in severe congenital and acquired valvular heart disease not as a last resort in prolonged vaginal delivery, complicated by heart failure, but as a preventive timely intervention.

Spontaneous vaginal delivery is possible in the absence of heart failure in patients with mitral regurgitation, predominant mitral stenosis in mixed mitral stenosis and regurgitation, aortic regurgitation or stenosis, and acyanotic congenital heart diseases.

Management of spontaneous (and surgical) labor in patients with heart diseases requires the participation of a cardiologist (internist) and an anesthesiologist. Anesthesia during labor is a preventive measure against heart failure development. It should be started with the first labor pains by intramuscular injection of 0.01 g diazepam (Valium) and 0.02 g pethidine (Vanina et al. 1977). There exists no consensus as to the type of anesthesia in patients with cardiovascular diseases. There are ardent proponents of epidural anesthesia (Metcalfe and Ueland 1978; Julian and Szekely 1985). It is indeed pain relieving, although it may sometimes cause an acute BP fall due to pronounced vasodilatation in the lower limbs. The procedure is to be performed by an experienced anesthesiologist under constant BP monitoring. This type of anesthesia constitutes the greatest threat in patients with pulmonary hypertension (secondary and primary), aortic stenosis (valvular and supravalvular), and hypertrophic cardiomyopathy in whom an additional reduction of the pregnancy-induced decrease in peripheral vascular resistance can give rise to severe collapse. This type of anesthesia should not be used in pregnant women on anticoagulants, as there is a risk of traumatic bleeding from major epidural veins. The vasodilating effect of epidural anesthesia can prove useful in heart failure. General anesthesia with halothane and other inhalation anesthetics with negative inotropic action has a favorable hemodynamic effect in patients with coarctation of the aorta, hypertrophic cardiomyopathy, and Marfan's syndrome, and an adverse hemodynamic effect in patients with mitral or aortic regurgitation. Spinal anesthesia, causing unpredictable hemodynamic shifts in patients with cardiovascular diseases, should not be used (Sullivan and Ramanathan 1985). In the absence of pulmonary hypertension or preeclampsia-eclampsia inhalation of pentothal (thiopental sodium)-nitrous oxide-oxygen mixture can be used. In patients with pulmonary hypertension and in those with threatening pulmonary edema, neuroleptanalgesia is recommended (Vanina et al. 1977). Fentanyl, having an adverse effect on the fetus, should be replaced by 0.02 g pethidine injected intramuscularly in combination with 2.5–5 mg droperidol. Hydroxydione sodium succinate injected intravenously (preferably into the vena cubitalis) proved useful in patients with cardiovascular disorders. There is evidence (Pavlova 1974; Pankratova 1974) that in using drugs one must take into account not only the woman's body weight but also the patient's functional class. In heart failure, class I, the drug dose should not exceed 8–9 mg/kg and in class II patients and class III–IV patients it should not exceed 7 mg/kg and 5–6 mg/kg, respectively. With almost complete cervical opening inhalation anesthesia is more advisable. Promethazine hydrochloride is also used. In forceps delivery and damaged tissue suturing, propanidid or nitrous oxide-oxygen mixture is used. Barbiturate and scopolamine adminstration should be avoided. Ether narcosis is contraindicated. In the presence of high arterial hypertension halothane anesthesia is advisable during surgical intervention (Pavlova 1974; Pankratova 1974). However, physicians should bear in mind that halothane may cause uterine relaxation, and attenuate the response to oxytocin and ergometrine injections. In addition, in abrupt blood pressure fall subsequent epinephrine or norepinephrine injections may give rise to severe arrhythmias.

The upper part of the body in women with heart disease should be tilted slightly upwards by raising the head end of the bed by 60–75 cm — Fowler's position. The legs should be supported below the level of the heart throughout the whole labor period to minimize venous return (Rush 1983). Nesbitt and Abdul-Karim (1982) believe it possible to keep women during labor in the dorsal lithotomic position for a short period. Oxygen therapy should be performed at times during the whole period of labor and delivery. Cardiac glycosides and antiarrhythmic agents are administered, if indicated. Preventive administration of antibiotics is recommended (Rush 1983), i.e., intravenous injections of 500 mg ampicillin 6 hourly and an aminoglycoside injection 8 hourly. Infusions of large volumes of drug solutions are not recommended because of a potential threat of pulmonary edema. If indicated, intravenous drip infusions should be carried out under careful control of venous blood pressure and the woman's condition. During labor, to reveal early signs of decompensation heart rate (not more than 110 beats/min) and breathing rate (not more than 24/min) should be monitored; blood pressure level and, if possible, cardiac output, acid-base balance, and PaO_2 should also be monitored. The condition of the fetus should be monitored by external cardiotocography.

It is necessary to watch the color of the skin (cyanosis indicates oxygen deficiency; severe pallor is a sign of vascular insufficiency) and to perform lung auscultation (congestive rales at lung bases may predict the development of pulmonary edema). If there are no contraindications (heart block) preventive intravenous injection of 0.025% digoxin or 0.5 ml 0.05% ouabain may be made in the first stage of labor, with the injection repeated in the puerperium. Some authors (Taurelle and Duhon 1976; etc.) recommend amniotomy and/or oxytocin injection as measures of heart failure prevention in the first stage of labor, which we do not believe advisable. First, amniotomy considerably delays the cervix opening and, second, oxytocin injection causes 300–500 ml deposited uterine blood to enter the vascular bed (De Swiet 1976), thus possibly inducing cardiac volume overload and critical pulmonary edema in patients with severe mitral stenosis. Amnion perforation precipitating labor is expedient only in an already dilated cervix. If it is still necessary to induce labor, patients with severe heart disease should not be placed in the lithotomic position to facilitate rupture of the membranes, as it is associated with unfavorable hemodynamic shifts.

At the second stage of labor in women with cardiovascular disorders (including patients who have undergone cardiac surgery) and in pregnant women with heart failure (even if the symptoms are relieved by the moment of labor) or with coronary insufficiency, it would be advisable, or even necessary to circumvent labor efforts by resorting to forceps delivery. Forceps are to be used under local, intravenous, or inhalation anesthesia. This measure diminishes the load on the cardiovascular system and shortens the second stage of labor. Well-timed episiotomy and/or perineotomy can to a certain extent contribute to the decrease of cardiovascular burden. Vacuum extraction instead of forceps delivery recommended by some authors (Conradsson and Werkö 1974; Kofler et al. 1982) seems less preferable since labor efforts are not completely relieved. The use of epidural anesthesia performed by skilled hands during forceps delivery and vacuum extraction advised by some authors is open to debate, though in patients with severe mitral stenosis this may promote blood deposition in the lower limbs and reduction of circulating blood volume, while pudendal and perineal anesthesia in such interventions can be used in patients showing no signs of heart failure.

In patients with implanted artificial pacemakers, possible dislocation of an intracardiac electrode cannot be excluded, and, therefore, one should be ready for emergency transvenous electrode insertion for temporary electrical stimulation.

Abdominal delivery is indicated in pregnancies complicated by heart failure (functional class III–IV) persisting until term; in active rheumatic carditis (glucocorticoid therapy, if it was started during pregnancy, should be continued both during labor and in the postoperative period); in severe mitral stenosis; bacterial endocarditis, coarctation of the aorta with high arterial hypertension or manifestations of beginning aortic dissection; in severe persistent atrial fibrillation; in extended myocardial infarction and deteriorated hemodynamics; and in heart disease and associated obstetric pathology. It should, however, be noted that there is a report on successful vaginal delivery in patients of functional class III–IV with mitral stenosis in the case of preload optimization by careful control of diuresis and heart rate regulation with propranolol (Clark et al. 1985). Cesarean section is contraindicated in severe pulmonary hypertension (including primary pulmonary hypertension).

The most suitable anesthetic management for cesarean section is inhalation anesthesia with neuroleptanalgesia and muscle relaxants. The method permits controlled respiration. Pulmonary artery pressure should be monitored with a flow-directed catheter, and direct measurements of arterial pressure should be performed. When there is a threat of severe heart failure, some authors (Metcalfe and Ueland 1974) recommend epidural anesthesia. Lumbar anesthesia is also possible (Sullivan and Ramanathan 1985). Prior to the operation the patients are given tranquilizers and those on glucocorticoids are orally administered 20 mg prednisolone. During operation 0.25–0.37 ml 0.05% ouabain is administered intravenously. During surgery of pregnant women with heart diseases Trendelenburg's position should be avoided, and immediately following the fetus extraction the head end of the operation table should be lifted. In threatening pulmonary edema venous tourniquets are applied to the thighs, with their relaxation started by the end of the operation and completed only when the operation is over. In impaired heart function this prevents rapid and undesirable redistribution of the blood. The postoperative period requires careful monitoring for fear of heart failure development. Therefore, preventive injection of cardiac glycosides seems expedient, though in recent years the efficacy of preventive therapy with cardiac glycosides has often been doubted. Analgesics, sedatives, as well as oxygen therapy and respiratory exercises are indicated.

Successful delivery in patients with severe congenital valvular heart disease is ensured in conditions of hyperbaric oxygenation (Burakovsky et al. 1976; Petrovsky et al. 1981).

To induce premature vaginal delivery in pregnant women with heart diseases estrogens are administered and cervix "maturity" is achieved, followed by amniotomy and intravenous infusion of oxytocin under constant monitoring of circulatory parameters. In recent years prostaglandins E_2 and $F_{2\alpha}$ administered orally, intravenously, or into the posterior fornix have been used to induce labor. As has already been mentioned in Chap. 1, the doses used do not have a significant effect on hemodynamics. If drug stimulation of labor causes the onset or increase of heart failure signs urgent abdominal delivery by cesarean section should be performed.

Immediately after spontaneous delivery, a load should be applied to the woman's abdomen. The fourth stage of labor and early puerperium in women with valvular heart diseases (particularly those accompanied by heart failure) are often complicated by uterine bleeding, which is arrested by oxytocin (5 units, intramuscularly) or methylergometrine injection. Though there exists a certain risk of systemic arterial pressure and pulmonary wedge pressure elevation (or in rare cases attacks in patients with Raynaud's disease), at present preventive injections of methylergometrine are often performed in the third stage of labor. This should be avoided in patients with heart disease predisposed to pulmonary wedge pressure elevation and in patients with arterial hypertension. However, it should be borne in mind that both methylergometrine and oxytocin administrations can sometimes promote the development of pulmonary edema. Patients at high risk of pulmonary edema (primarily those with mitral stenosis) should be injected 20 mg furosemide intravenously immediately before methylergometrine or oxytocin administration. Pulmonary edema can also develop when during collapse caused by blood loss (such collapse predominates in patients with septal defects) excessive amounts of blood expanders are given or pressor amines are administered in large volumes of a 5% glucose or other isotonic solutions. When blood loss compensation is required isogroup blood transfusion is preferable and in cases of hypofibrinogenemia fibrinogen or dry blood plasma should be administered.

Postpartal hemodynamic adjustment occurs mainly in the first 48 (sometimes 72) h after delivery. In this period the condition of women with cardiovascular disease, especially those at high risk of pulmonary edema, should be carefully followed. Right ventricular, left ventricular, and total heart failure, pulmonary thromboembolism, collapse, rheumatic fever recurrence, and pyogenic and inflammatory diseases (mastitis, endomyometritis, thrombophlebitis, etc.) can possibly develop. In view of the above, preventive and therapeutic measures seem necessary. If no heart failure was detected in the prepregnancy period or during pregnancy and labor, 1 week bed rest will suffice for women with heart disease. Some authors (Metcalfe and Ueland 1974; Taurelle and Duhon 1976) speak in favor of early postpartum mobilization of patients with heart diseases, with Kunz and Zogg (1980) beginning mobilization of patients in good condition already on the 2nd day after delivery. Early standing and walking in the puerperium, as well as using carefully fitted elastic stockings, considerably decrease the risk of thromboembolism (Metcalfe and Ueland 1978; Rush 1983). If a puerpera has had heart failure in her history, during labor, or in the postpartal period she must be kept in bed for 2–3 weeks. With persistent heart failure and in the absence of postdelivery obstetric complications 3–4 weeks after delivery, the patient should be transported to a cardiological department of a hospital.

Prevention of thromboembolic complications in the puerperium may pose a serious problem in patients with Eisenmenger's syndrome, primary pulmonary hypertension, and other heart lesions predisposing to thromboembolism. Heparin therapy, necessary in such cases, may promote postpartal bleedings, while discontinuation of such therapy sometimes leads to cerebral embolism and death. And still, heparin therapy for 1–2 weeks after labor seems advisable in these cases for thrombosis prevention. Gradual replacement of heparin by oral anticoagulants is possible.

There is no consensus as to whether preventive antibiotic therapy of bacterial endocarditis is necessary (in women with heart disease) following normal delivery. Some authors (De Swiet 1976; Kunz and Zogg 1980) consider it obligatory, while others (Sugrue et al. 1980; Nesbitt and Abdul-Karim 1982; Kofler et al. 1982; Deeg 1983) believe it unnecessary. Prevention of bacterial endocarditis seems advisable in pregnant women with prosthetic cardiac valves (Casanegra et al. 1975) and obligatory after manual separation of the placenta, cesarean section, or abortion. To prevent endocarditis intramuscular injections of up to 20 million units of penicillin and 80 mg gentamicin or intramuscular or intravenous injections of 1 g ampicillin are recommended 30 min prior to manual separation of the placenta. In cases of penicillin intolerance 1 g intravenous vancomycin and 1 g intramuscular streptomycin would suffice. Preventive administration of antibiotics in heart disease threatened with the onset of endocarditis should be continued 4–6 days after labor (Szekely and Snaith 1974).

Tocolysis is another obstetric intervention which should be performed with consideration of heart disease. A betamimetic fenoterol commonly used for the prevention of premature labor along with the ability to depress uterine contractions has a positive inotropic and chronotropic effect. This may create an unfavorable hemodynamic situation in pregnant women with mitral and aortic stenosis, hypertrophic cardiomyopathy, myocarditis, and some forms of congenital heart disease, leading in some cases to pulmonary edema or supraventricular or ventricular arrhythmias (Deeg 1983). This drug should be used with utmost caution. An undesirable effect of fenoterol may be attenuated by cardioselective beta-blockers, lacking intrinsic sympathomimetic activity (atenolol, metoprolol, at a dose of 50–100 mg), or calcium antagonists (verapamil at a dose of 80–120 mg/day) (Deeg 1983). Aminophylline, indomethacin, and flufenamic acid all possess tocolytic activity and seem to be the drugs of choice.

There is also a problem concerning the newborn. The use of aspirin (prolonging the labor period and increasing the risk of bleeding in the mother and newborn), benzodiazepines (leading to neonatal withdrawal syndrome), methyldopa (inducing neonatal meconium ileus), and reserpine (increasing the secretion of respiratory tract epithelium in the newborn and causing nasal congestion and anorexia) should, if possible, be discontinued before labor.

Anticoagulant therapy should also be performed with caution. To reduce the risk of bleeding at the beginning and in anticipation of labor, heparin should be discontinued and protamine sulfate should be injected — this moment is especially easy to establish in labor induction (Perloff 1984). If spontaneous labor begins in a patient on coumarin anticoagulants, frozen plasma administration (McCans and Wenger 1976) and oxytocin drip infusion (Kofler et al. 1982) are advisable. If cesarean section is planned in advance in such a patient the anticoagulants should be withdrawn 2–3 days before the intervention (Ibarra-Perez et al. 1976). A day after labor anticoagulant therapy is to be resumed.

11.2 Breast Feeding and Drugs

Breast feeding does not aggravate the condition of women with cardiovascular disorders, except for patients with congestive heart failure (NYHA functional class III and IV), in whom lactation should be suppressed.

One must be aware of the fact that some drugs can enter breast milk. The amounts of drugs entering breast milk are not always high enough to affect the newborn. However, there are diverse opinions as to the risk of this or that drug for children of breast-feeding mothers. Therefore, the physician should make a decision considering all the "pros" and "cons". The data (often conflicting) on the effect of drugs entering breast milk on the newborn are summarized in the works by Soradi (1980), Kunz and Schreiner (1982), Pepperell (1983), Berglund et al. (1984), and Lauritzen (1985).

Penicillin and its derivatives are harmless for the newborn (though in rare cases skin allergic reactions can occur). Tetracycline derivatives can cause staining of the baby's tooth enamel, growth delay, and changes in the intestinal flora spectrum (disbacteriosis), while chloramphenicol can cause infantile jaundice and disbacteriosis. Therefore, drugs of the above-mentioned groups must not be given to nursing mothers. Streptomycin enters breast wilk in very small quantities and is harmless for the baby, as well as erythromycin, lincomycin, and kanamycin. The use of sulfonamides has the risk of causing nuclear jaundice. Isoquinoline drugs [Plaquenil (hydroxychloroquine sulfate), chloroquine, etc.] can cause moderate thrombocytopenia in the newborn. Salicylates should be given in moderate doses, as they are capable of causing jaundice, respiratory disorders, acidosis, and thrombocytopenia. Phenylbutazone can be given to nursing mothers as it enters breast milk in small concentrations. Barbituric acid derivatives as hypnotic agents should not be given to nursing mothers, for they easily enter breast milk, having an adverse effect on the newborn. Chlordiazepoxide, diazepam, and antihistamine agents, entering breast milk in very small quantities, are harmless for the newborn; however, their long-term use by nursing mothers is inadvisable. Coumarin agents taken by the mother in some cases cause hemorrages in the baby, while heparin, whose amounts in breast milk are negligible, is safe. Cardiac glycosides, epinephrine, norepinephrine, and furosemide are used in the treatment of nursing mothers. Hydrochlorothiazide, like other thiazide diuretics, can cause hypokalemia and thrombocytopenia in the newborn. Corticosteroids easily enter breast milk and can cause neonatal jaundice. Propranolol can reduce heart rate and cardiac output in the newborn. Sotalol and timolol content in milk is rather high, and, therefore, they should be avoided. Iodine preparations can induce hypothyroidism and skin manifestations of iodism, while other thyrostatic agents cause hypothyroid goiter. The effect of atropine that the baby gets via its mother's milk is unknown, and, therefore, it is safer to avoid its use throughout the lactation period. Chlorthalidone and furosemide have been reported to suppress lactation and thus their long-term use or administration in high doses is inadvisable.

Drug administration to nursing mothers is performed only when strictly indicated and with regard to possible drug effect on the baby; long-term treatment, if required should be carried out at intervals. When it is necessary to administer agents that are harmful for the newborns, breast feeding should be stopped.

11.3 Termination of Pregnancy in Patients with Cardiovascular Diseases

Termination of pregnancy in women with heart diseases requires the patient's pretreatment (sedative, cardiotonic, antirheumatic therapy) and careful analgesia (in severe conditions — inhalation nitrous oxide-oxygen anesthesia). Up to 12 weeks of gestation common or suction curettage is used; later in pregnancy cesarean section is performed with the patient under anesthesia. At present, to terminate pregnancies, intraamniotic, extraamniotic, intravenous, and intramuscular injections of prostaglandin $F_{2\alpha}$ or its synthetic analogue — 15-methylprostaglandin $F_{2\alpha}$ — are successfully used in weeks 13–27 of gestation. As such abortions take little time and the doses of prostaglandin used do not have a pronounced effect on the heart muscle and hemodynamics, this method of pregnancy termination is recommended in patients with heart diseases (Persianinov et al. 1978; Samoylova et al. 1979). However, there are authors who object to the use of prostaglandin $F_{2\alpha}$, which has a vasoconstrictive effect in patients with cardiovascular diseases (Rush 1983; Chard and Lilford 1983). Extraamniotic administration of hypertonic salt or other solutions to induce premature labor in pregnant women with heart disease is inadmissible. If a women with a valvular heart disease already has children and the heart disease is surgically incurable it is advisable to recommend her tube ligation. The procedure should be carried out via the abdominal approach (a laparoscope is not to be used, as pregnant women with heart diseases poorly endure pneumoperitoneum).

Termination of pregnancy in women with heart disease can sometimes worsen the patient's hemodynamic state, with various extracardiac complications sometimes developing after the intervention. Thus, women with heart diseases in whom pregnancy is undesirable or dangerous should be recommended either thorough contraception or sterilization.

12 Hypertension and Pregnancy

Elevated blood pressure in pregnancy may be a manifestation of different diseases: essential hypertension, renal artery stenosis or occlusion, chronic glomerulonephritis or pyelonephritis (sometimes in combination with nephrolithiasis), coarctation of the aorta, pheochromocytoma, Conn's syndrome, Cushing's syndrome, preeclampsia, and a number of uncommon diseases, as well as diabetic nephropathy. Differential diagnosis of these diseases in pregnancy is associated with some difficulties; and, in addition, preeclampsia may be superimposed on any diseases characterized by high blood pressure. Since the diagnostic criteria and statistical data of different authors are heterogeneous, it is difficult to indicate the true incidence of each of these diseases in pregnancy. For instance, some authors tend to consider any elevation of blood pressure in the second half of pregnancy a sign of preeclampsia, while others even in the presence of the classical triad of preeclampsia (hypertension, edema, albuminuria) suspect exacerbation of latent glomerulonephritis.

A blood pressure level above 140/90 mmHg is detected in 5%–20% of pregnant women (Foidart and Rorive 1977; Galleri et al. 1977). Hypertension can in some cases pose a vital threat to the mother. Murnaghan (1982) and Zuspan (1984) have reported that the decrease in the maternal mortality rate due to all causes has made hypertensive complications in pregnancy the most frequent cause of maternal death in some countries. Hypertension is sometimes the cause of placental detachment, premature labor, growth retardation, and even fetal death (Cibilis 1974; Finnerty 1977; Chervenak and Berkowitz 1985). However, the maternal prognosis is usually favorable if the first 20 weeks of gestation were not marked by a BP elevation above 160/100 mmHg (Snaith and Szekely 1974) and in the absence of renal failure or severe preeclampsia or eclampsia. According to the epidemiological data of Dequiedt et al. (1984), there are many patients with excess weight, hypercholesterolemia, essential hypertension, or diabetes mellitus in the history among pregnant women with arterial hypertension. Many of them used estrogen-progestagen contraceptive pills in the prepregnancy period. Hypertension is the most frequent reason for hospitalization of pregnant women in the antepartal period (Murnaghan 1982). Wellen (1953) reported that pregnant women with high blood pressure in 70% of cases have preeclampsia, in 15%–25% of the cases essential hypertension, and in the rest of cases secondary hypertension. However, according to the records of a specialized clinic, where pregnant women with definite or suspected preeclampsia were admitted, the incidence of "pure" preeclampsia ranked third after essential hypertension and the hypertensive form of pyelonephritis, combinations of preeclampsia with pyelonephritis, and essential hypertension being much less frequent (Finnerty 1977).

12.1 Essential Hypertension

Essential hypertension is a most widespread form of hypertension. Blood pressure elevation is the primary clinical sign. While in secondary hypertension high blood pressure is caused by primary lesions of kidneys, adrenal glands, aorta, and renal arteries, in essential hypertension damage of internal organs (namely, heart and kidneys) is secondary. It is generally accepted that essential hypertension results from impaired function of the central and autonomic nervous system mechanisms controlling blood pressure, and from shifts in the function of humoral pressure-regulating systems (renin-angiotensin-aldosterone, kallikrein-kinin, prostaglandins). Great etiological importance is attached to neuropsychic overstrain, psychoemotional traumas, prolonged exposure to negative emotions, unfavorable heredity, etc. Excessive salt and alcohol consumption and smoking can also play a certain role.

Pathogenetically blood pressure elevation is caused by disorders in the central nervous system and the sympathetic part of the autonomic nervous system, leading to the increase in cardiac output and, occasionally, circulating blood volume (in initial phases), the main reason being the rise in peripheral vascular resistance (mostly at the arteriolar level). Sodium excess-induced electrolyte imbalance in the vascular wall results in increased sensitivity of vascular smooth muscles to humoral pressor agents (angiotensin, catecholamines, etc.). Vascular wall swelling and thickening worsen blood supply of internal organs in spite of blood pressure elevation, with subsequent damage of the heart, kidneys, brain, and other organs resulting from arteriolar sclerosis. The heart, forced to overcome raised peripheral vascular resistance, becomes hypertrophied and in advanced stages dilated, which in the end can contribute to the onset of heart failure. Damage of small renal arteries and arterioles leads to renal ischemia, growth of juxtaglomerular apparatus, further activation of the renin-angiotensin system, and blood pressure stabilization at a higher level. Later, renal lesions are manifested in the decline of the glomerular filtration rate, and sometimes chronic renal failure can develop. Due to cerebral vessel damage patients with essential hypertension often develop hemorrhagic, sometimes fatal, stroke. Such severe cardiac, renal and cerebral lesions in women of childbearing age occur only in the case of severe and long-standing arterial hypertension as well as in malignant hypertension.

The disease has different stages. According to the WHO classification three stages are indentified.

Stage I: No objective signs of organic changes are evident.

Stage II: At least one of the following signs of organ involvement is present:

- Left ventricular hypertrophy on physical examination, chest X-ray, electrocardiography, echocardiography, etc.
- Generalized and focal narrowing of the retinal arteries.
- Proteinuria and/or slight elevation of plasma creatinine concentration.

Stage III: Both symptoms and signs have appeared as a result of damage to various organs from hypertensive disease. These include:

— Heart: left ventricular failure.
— Brain: cerebral, cerebellar, or brain stem hemorrage; hypertensive encephalopathy.
— Optic fundi: retinal hemorrhages and exudates with or without papilloedema. These features are pathognomonic of the malignant (accelerated) phase.

According to the predominant clinical syndrome, three forms of essential hypertension may be distinguished: cardiac (including coronary), renal, and cerebral.

Primary diagnosis of essential hypertension in pregnancy often poses certain difficulties. The majority of pregnant women with essential hypertension have elevated blood pressure in their history. However, it should be recognized that in some patients high blood pressure remains practically unchanged during pregnancy, while in others it increases, and in some it normalizes or falls below the normal level. An increase in the elevated prepregnancy blood pressure level can be mediated by superimposed preeclampsia with the appearance of edema (mostly insignificant) and/or albuminuria. Temporary blood pressure decrease in patients with essential hypertension is commonly observed in the first or second trimester, with blood pressure elevation occurring again in the third trimester of pregnancy or in the puerperium (Eliseev 1979; Finnerty 1980). In the absence of essential hypertension in the history BP elevation in the third trimester of pregnancy complicates differential diagnosis between essential hypertension and preeclampsia.

When the history is not clear, essential hypertension can be suspected by a positive familial history of arterial hypertension, early blood pressure elevation (before the 20th week of gestation) with no concomitant edema and albuminuria or with insignificant albuminuria, the relatively advanced age of the patient, retinal angiosclerosis, left ventricular hypertrophy, and data on blood pressure elevation during previous pregnancies (preeclampsia is less frequent in repeated pregnancies).

Pregnant women with arterial hypertension show some specific pregnancy-induced hemodynamic changes. Cardiac index and blood volume increases in such cases are less marked (Smith et al. 1967) and plasma volume is considerably lower (Hunyor 1984) than in normal pregnancies. During blood pressure elevation renal and uterine blood flow reduces (Pontonier et al. 1975; Shekhtman and Glezer 1978).

Pregnant women with essential hypertension are often asymptomatic. In some cases the prevailing complaints are: easy fatigability, sleep disturbances, headaches (more often occipital), dizziness, and flickering in the eyes; less frequently the patients complain of epistaxis, palpitation, stabbing chest pain, and numbness of fingers. The examination can reveal systolic murmur at the heart apex and sometimes at the aortic area; accentuated aortic component of the second heart sound can be also heard. The pulse is hyperkinetic. Both systolic and diastolic arterial pressures are raised.

Roentgenographic findings reveal left ventricular hypertrophy, and slight lengthening and tortuosity of the aorta. ECG findings of left ventricular hypertrophy are as follows: leftward rotation of the electrical heart axis, R wave and S wave amplitude increase in leads $V_{5,6}$ and $V_{1,2}$, respectively (the sum of the amplitudes of the highest R wave and the deepest S wave exceeding 45 mm), and moderate widening of the QRS complex. As ventricular hypertrophy advances, ST segment depression and T wave flattening (and later inversion) in leads $V_{5,6}$ occur. Echocardiography reveals an increase in left ventricular mass (as compared with that observed in normotensive pregnant women) even in moderate and newly developed BP elevation (Hunyor 1984). Hypertensive retinopathy is often found. In some cases insignificant albuminuria and single erythrocytes are noted in the urine. Renal blood flow is already reduced in the early stages of the disease.

The course of essential hypertension is sometimes characterized by crises, accompanied by severe headaches. In early stages of the disease the crises last 1–3 h and are accompanied by anxiety, tremor, enhanced perspiration, tachycardia, and sometimes stabbing chest pain. Such a crisis was termed type I crisis (Ratner 1974) and is characterized predominantly by systolic pressure increase. Type II crises are seen in patients with essential hypertension, stage II and III. They can last 3–4 days and are more severe than type I crises, demonstrating mostly neurological symptoms (hypertensive encephalopathy). The signs of hypertensive encephalopathy (severe headache, nausea, vomiting, dizziness, often peculiar drowsiness) are similar to those of preeclamptic encephalopathy. Type II crises are sometimes characterized by transient disturbances of cerebral blood flow and vision, and the onset of left ventricular heart failure. If the blood pressure is high, cerebral hemorrhages (mainly during labor) can be fatal. However, transitory disturbances of cerebral blood flow are more frequently observed, particularly in premature labor. If examinations of pregnant women with essential hypertension are regular and their treatment adequate, such complications are rare (Eliseev 1979).

Maternal prognosis in the majority of cases is favorable. In 85% of pregnant women with uncomplicated essential hypertension the disease course is not aggravated. In high stable hypertension uteroplacental circulation is impaired, which often results in fetal hypotrophy. Sometimes pregnant women with essential hypertension have premature labor. Superimposed preeclampsia in pateints with essential hypertension poses a threat to both mother and fetus, for it is associated with increased risk of stillbirth, premature labor, placental separation, acute renal failure, and maternal death. Superimposed preeclampsia in hypertensive patients with pronounced left ventricular dilation and considerable electrocardiographic changes is associated with a high risk of heart failure. With a maternal diastolic blood pressure of 120 mmHg and higher, the perinatal mortality rate is considerably increased. The prognosis is poor for pregnant women who have had essential hypertension complicated by preeclampsia during previous pregnancy.

It is difficult to identify the true incidence of cases in which essential hypertension is complicated by preeclampsia, for the diagnostic criteria vary from author to author. According to Chesley (1978), it is 5.7% using strict criteria, but the author himself believes it to be higher. Shekhtman and Barkhatova (1982) hold that superimposed preeclampsia occurs in 36% of pregnant women with essential hypertension. Perloff (1984) believes that moderate essential hypertension is complicated by preeclampsia in 10%–20% of cases and then BP elevated in early pregnancy rises considerably in the third trimester of gestation. Perinatal mortality, when these two pathological conditions are combined, is sure to be several times higher than perinatal mortality of women suffering from essential hypertension alone.

Malignant arterial hypertension is rare in pregnant women, though it prevails in relatively young persons. This form of the disease is characterized by stable blood pressure elevation unresponding to routine treatment, papilloedema, exudation and hemorrhages on the eyegrounds, signs of renal failure, cerebral circulation disorders, and heart failure. Pregnancy drastically aggravates the course of the disease, especially promoting renal failure that can lead to death of uremia. In spite of pregnancy, body weight in these patients decreases as well as the glomerular filtration rate. Early stillbirths with following (in several weeks or months) maternal death are typical. Death also usually occurs several months after therapeutic abortion.

Pregnancy is contraindicated in malignant arterial hypertension and in essential hypertension, stage III. If the first weeks and months of gestation are characterized by stable blood pressure elevation, marked left ventricular hypertrophy and serious eyeground changes, the risk of preeclampsia in later pregnancy is very high. It increases still further when there is a concomitant impairment of renal function. Such refractory hypertension accompanied by organic changes is an indication for the termination of pregnancy (Sokolow and McIlroy 1981).

12.2 Preeclampsia-Eclampsia

In spite of a considerable fall in the death rate from eclampsia it continues to be among the important causes of maternal and fetal mortality. This may, to some extent, be attributable to the lack of definite knowledge on its causes and mechanisms, making prevention and treatment of the condition difficult. Neither the etiology nor the pathogenesis of preeclampsia-eclampsia are known for certain. The true incidence of these variously named pathological conditions (preeclampsia, toxemia of pregnancy, late gestosis, pregnancy-induced hypertension) is difficult to determine because of differences in definition and criteria. The data reported in various sources vary from 1%–2% to 25%–30% (Lindmark et al. 1984). Preeclampsia was observed in 5%–10% of pregnancies, including cases when it accompanied arterial hypertension of different origin (Sokolow and McIlroy 1981; Lindmark et al. 1984), with its incidence gradually decreasing in the most recent decades. Eclampsia is much less frequent, being encountered in about 0.1% of pregnant women; but the maternal mortality rate from eclampsia stands at 5%–14% (Speroff 1973; Sokolow and McIlroy 1981) and fetal mortality at 15%–30% (Speroff 1973; Perloff 1984). Preeclampsia is more frequent in hypertensive patients, in pregnant women with preeclampsia or eclampsia in their history, in patients with diabetes mellitus, renal diseases, and hydatiform mole, in primigravidas, and in twin pregnancies.

In recent years an essential role in the pathogenesis of preeclampsia has been attributed to the immunological conflict (IgG and IgM, as well as C_3 complement component were detected in the kidneys) between the mother, placenta, and fetus (Suc et al. 1978; Takeda et al. 1985), as well as to adrenal mineralocorticoid function disorder and intravascular coagulation (caused by trophoblast emboli or thromboplastin, produced during trophoblast degeneration) with fibrin depositions in arterial walls of the liver and particularly the kidneys (Howie et al. 1976; Takeda et al. 1985) and pathognomonic damage of renal glomeruli, whose endothelial cells expose phagocytic activity and absorb fibrin. The intracapillary cell swelling and vacuolization with the narrowing of glomerular capillary lumen was found in preeclampsia (Spargo et al. 1976). The percentage of polymorphonuclear leukocytes and platelets whose surface membranes are bound to IgG, IgM, IgA, and C_3 is considerably higher in pregnant women with preeclampsia than in healthy pregnant and nonpregnant women. In severe preeclampsia, the C_3 complement component content is considerably increased. The level of circulating immune complexes is elevated; however, this might also be observed in normal pregnancy (Massobrio et al. 1985). The studies by Wohlhert et al. (1984) have also shown that circulating immune complexes in pregnancy cannot serve as signs of either preeclampsia or essential hypertension.

Placental ischemia plays an essential role in the pathogenesis of eclampsia. Acute rise of intrauterine pressure or acute decrease of uterine blood flow result in blood pressure elevation in experimental animals obviously aimed at the recovery of utero-placental circulation. A chronic experiment (Cavanagh et al. 1972) applying blood flow limiting clamps to uterine arteries and performing ovarian artery ligation showed the development of proteinuria and hypertension in the third trimester of pregnancy in monkeys. The clinical importance of placental ischemia is confirmed by the higher incidence of preeclampsia in young primiparas (with somewhat hypoplastic uterus), multiple pregnancy, hydroamnion, hydatidiform mole, and essential hypertension (i.e., hypertension-mediated placental ischemia). Finally, placental ischemia can become the cause of embolism with trophoblast products in different vascular regions. Enhanced vasoconstriction and platelet aggregation may be associated with the fact that, unlike normal pregnancy, in preeclampsia the placenta produces nonequivalent amounts of thromboxane and prostacyclin, with thromboxane production exceeding prostacyclin production seven fold (Walsh 1985). In addition, the enhanced reaction of resistive vessels, isolated from the omentum, to angiotensin II has been observed in preeclampsia (Aalkjaer et al. 1985). The presumptive role of humoral pressor agents (hysperotonin, peptides from the placenta, trophoblast, amniotic fluid, decidual membrane) or deficiency of vasodilating substances (prostaglandins A and E) of trophoblastic or renal origin in the pathogenesis of hypertension in preeclampsia has not yet been proved (Pirani and McGillivray 1975; Foidart and Rorive 1977), though interesting data on prostaglandin E have recently been obtained. Its level in healthy pregnant women doubles, while in pregnant women with nonpreeclamptic hypertension its level increases threefold, as compared with normal. In preeclampsia its level remains practically normal (Kovatz et al. 1985). Placental dysfunction is sure to play a certain role in the pathogenesis of preeclampsia; it disappears after placental rejection.

Blood pressure elevation in pregnant women with preeclampsia is caused by an increase in peripheral vascular resistance, associated with enhanced reactivity of arteriolar smooth muscle fibers (observed several weeks prior to clinical symptoms and signs of preeclampsia). It should be noted that the increase in peripheral vascular resistance in preeclampsia is not related to the enhanced activity of the sympathetic part of the autonomic nervous system; that is why ganglioblockers (to which pregnant women with essential hypertension are so sensitive) and even spinal anesthesia have practically no effect on the blood pressure level (Assali and Brinkman 1972). The rise in peripheral vascular resistance is not related to the increase in renin-angiotensin-aldosterone system activity. Blood plasma renin activity and angiotensinogen, angiotensin II, and aldosterone levels are lower in preeclampsia than in normal pregnancy (Weir et al. 1973). Therefore, it is difficult to account for sodium retention in pregnant women with preeclampsia, which in other diseases is mostly associated with increased renin-angiotensin-aldosterone system activity. However, kallikrein excretion, considerably increased in normal pregnancy and pregnant patients with essential hypertension, is reduced by half (as compared with normal) in pregnant women with preeclampsia (Kovatz et al. 1985). Thus, kallikrein system dysfunction may play a certain role.

The increase in sodium excretion following salt load is expressed less in preeclampsia than in patients with essential hypertension. Sodium retention in the body is more pronounced in preeclampsia than in normal pregnancy, with the degree of water retention according to Little (1965) somewhat exceeding the degree of sodium retention, while according to other authors, the degree of sodium retention is, on the contrary, more pronounced than the degree of water retention. Strange as it may seem, in preeclampsia sodium load and high sodium diet are sometimes well tolerated (Mengert and Tacehi 1961).

Preeclampsia usually develops following the 20th–26th week of pregnancy and is more frequent in primigravidas than in multigravidas; the earlier preeclampsia occurs, the greater the risk for the mother and fetus (Lin et al. 1982). Besides, marked arterial hypertension, upper body edema (periorbital and arm edema) and proteinuria (not less than 3 g/liter) commonly developing upon BP elevation and the onset of edema (Finnerty 1980) are typical clinical signs of preeclampsia. However, these signs are not always equally pronounced, sometimes one or even two of them may be absent. Preeclampsia and even eclampsia are, in rare cases, accompanied by "normal" blood pressure, i.e., when blood pressure in women suffering from arterial hypotension increases by 20–30 mmHg, not exceeding the upper normal limit (Eliseev 1981).

The patients usually complain of a heavy feeling in the head, headache, dyspnea, and visual disturbances. Bradycardia and heart rhythm disorders can be observed occasionally. Left ventricular hypertrophy is not usually found, unless it was caused by a disease preceding preeclampsia. ECG in many patients with preeclampsia shows ST segment and T wave changes, sometimes associated with notched QRS complex. All these disorders are considered to be manifestations of toxemic cardiomyopathy (Burch 1977), which aggravates the prognosis, the remote one included. Blood pressure elevation is at first somewhat unstable; however, as the disease develops, it reaches a very high level, especially in eclampsia. Circadian blood pressure fluctuations are less marked in patients with preeclampsia than in pregnant women with essential hypertension (Eliseev 1981). Eyeground examination reveals angiospastic retinopathy.

Not only such signs as BP elevation and the development or the increase of proteinuria, but also visual disturbances, rapid weight gain, and noticeable reduction in diuresis should put the physician on guard. Water retention in preeclampsia varies from covert edema to anasarca. The urine specific weight is high. Urine protein content may also be high, but its most usual level does not exceed 3–6 g/liter. Few cylinders are found in urinary sediment. The glomerular filtration rate can be decreased, with tubular reabsorption remaining normal. Examination of the blood often reveals marked hypoproteinemia, and increased level of blood urea nitrogen. Plasma volume is reduced and hematocrit is raised. In excessive sodium and water intake acute heart failure can develop accompanied by pulmonary edema, especially in the presence of renal dysfunction.

Symptoms and signs of preeclampsia and eclampsia are largely conditioned by the disorders of the central nervous system, associated with cerebral blood flow disturbances. Symptoms of preeclampsia are: headache, visual disturbances, drowsiness, epigastric pain, and sometimes nausea, vomiting, abdominal pain, and diarrhea. Severe cases are accompanied by excitement.

Eclampsia (sometimes following attacks of severe headaches) is manifested in tonic and clonic 1- to 3-min-long convulsions, followed by comatose state. The fit begins with minute fibrillar twitching of facial muscles, quickly involving the upper limbs and the muscles of the whole body. The fit is accompanied by respiratory arrest, slowing heart rate, and further blood pressure elevation. Eclampsia episodes can lead to death of asphyxia with cardiac arrest or of acute pulmonary edema. It can also result in possibly fatal cerebral hemorrhages. Bauer et al. (1982) have observed contraction band necrosis secondary to coronary reperfusion upon blood flow arrest in about one-third of the patients who died of eclampsia, which suggests a high incidence of coronary spasm in these patients. In rare cases, eclampsia is not preceded by blood pressure elevation, edema, and albuminuria. Convulsions can also occur during labor and very seldom in the puerperium. Complications of eclampsia are as follows: (a) disseminated intravascular coagulation with profuse bleeding; (b) capillary leak syndrome with severe proteinuria, serous effusions, and acute pulmonary edema; (c) intrahepatic hemorrhages, infarctions, and even liver rupture; and (d) acute renal failure caused by acute tubular or cortical necrosis (Lubbe 1984). The prognosis in preeclampsia is poor when it develops prior to the 30th week of gestation, is long-standing, and is refractory to therapy.

At present, severe preeclampsia and eclampsia are rare and the maternal mortality of eclampsia (to be more exact of its hypertension-induced complications, primarily of cerebral hemorrhages) is relatively low. However, arterial hypertension related to preeclampsia is still a frequent cause of premature placental separation, premature delivery, fetal hypoxia, growth retardation, and death. The long-term prognosis for years ahead differs significantly in women with eclampsia in their history of the first or subsequent pregnancies. Seventy percent of primiparas are not exposed to increased risk of hypertension stabilization and cardiovascular death. Multiparas show a trend toward hypertension stabilization, and their cardiovascular mortality is three times higher than in women of the appropriate age group (Chesley et al. 1976).

It is essential that stable arterial hypertension remains in 20%–30% of women following preeclampsia. Sometimes it is the consequence of secondary nephropathy, i.e., activation of the preexisting latent chronic renal diseases (glomerulo- or pyelonephritis). In a fewer number of cases (however, according to some authors in 50% of cases) such hypertension results from specific primary nephropathy, histologically similar to the membranous form of glomerulonephritis. Sometimes a greater degree of glomerular endothelium damage, more pronounced dystrophic changes of tubular epithelium, and proliferation of mesangial cells are found, as compared with glomerulonephritis. Characteristic changes of juxtaglomerular apparatus cells and the basal membrane are shown in this form of nephropathy (Spargo et al. 1959; Altchek et al. 1968). And, finally, in certain cases, this so-called residual hypertension appears to result from the transitory form of essential hypertension turning into the stable one (Eliseev 1979).

12.3 Renovascular Hypertension

Renovascular hypertension is mediated by partial obstruction of one or sometimes both main renal arteries. Obstruction in women of childbearing age is mainly caused by fibromuscular hyperplasia of one or both (in one-third of cases) renal arteries, with the dystrophic sclerotic process impairing mostly arterial media and adventitia and periarterial fibrosis and intimal hyperplasia simultaneously developing. It results in the formation of stenosis sites and aneurysmic bulges. A charateristic angiographic pattern of the vessel is "goose throat" or "a string of beads". In some cases the damage is single focal. Sometimes not only the main renal artery is impaired but also its branches of the first and second order.

The second cause of renovascular hypertension in women of childbearing age is nonspecific aortoarteritis (Takayasu's disease), when there is a collagenosis-like (autoimmune) process selectively damaging the aortic arch and its major branches, and if the abdominal aorta is involved — also the proximal part of the renal arteries. The damage is usually bilateral. The process can be complicated by thrombosis of the renal artery. Hypertension can often assume a malignant course.

Though renovascular hypertension caused by a considerable stenosis of the ostium of one (or both) renal arteries by an atherosclerotic plaque may sometimes be found in patients under 40, it is an extremely rare case in women of childbearing age. Poststenotic dilation of the renal artery is usually distal to the stenosis site.

Renal ischemia, stimulating renin secretion and thus causing activation of the renin-angiotensin-aldosterone system, plays a decisive role in the pathogenesis of renovascular hypertension. Therefore, surgical elimination of arterial stenosis or percutaneous transluminal balloon dilation of the renal artery can result in the removal of renal ischemia and blood pressure normalization.

Patients with renovascular hypertension (in spite of a pronounced blood pressure elevation) are either asymptomatic or their complaints are identical to those of patients with essential hypertension. Blood pressure elevation is stable and often responds poorly to medication. Sometimes predominantly diastolic pressure is raised. High-frequency systolic or continuous vascular murmur, auscultated above the area of origin of the affected renal artery from the aorta. is the clinical sign of renovascular hypertension. No changes are usually found in the urine, except for occasional insignificant proteinuria.

It is difficult to diagnose renovascular hypertension in pregnancy, as aortography, radionuclide renography (revealing assymetry of renal function), radionuclide renal scanning, and intravenous urography (revealing the reduced size of one of the kidneys and relatively higher concentration of the contrast medium in it) are not to be performed during pregnancy, and the invasive study of differential renal excretory function and renin activity in renal venous plasma, though giving the most reliable data, are also inadvisable in pregnant women. The incidence of renovascular hypertension in hypertensive pregnant women is not known for certain.

Pregnancy is usually considered contraindicated in Takayasu's disease; however, several cases of successful delivery in women with this disease have been reported. Wang et al. (1982) reported an uncomplicated pregnancy and delivery in 15 patients with Takayasu's disease.

12.4 Primary Aldosteronism (Conn's Disease)

The disease is caused by an aldosterone-producing tumor (or hyperplasia) in the glomerular zone of the adrenal cortex and is accompanied by potassium loss, sodium retention, alkalosis, and hypertension. The incidence of the disease is higher in women. Aldosteroma (or adrenocortical hyperplasia) can be bilateral.

The patients complain of headache, dizziness, paresthesias, tetanic manifestations, transitory or stable muscle weakness, intermittent paralysis, polydipsia, nocturia, and polyuria. Examination reveals moderate (occasionally pronounced) blood pressure elevation, metabolic alkalosis, hypokalemia, decreased plasma renin activity, and increased urinary potassium and aldosterone excretion. The urine is usually alkaline, with low specific weight; often moderate proteinuria is noted. X-ray findings are left ventricular hypertrophy. QRS complex widening, ST segment depression, flat (sometimes diphasic) T wave, and U wave appearance (more marked in right chest leads) are observed in the ECG. In more severe cases, heart sounds are muffled, and premature beats, tachycardia, and occasional AV conduction disturbances are noted. One should be aware that in some cases the plasma potassium level may be normal in spite of its intracellular deficiency. Urinary aldosterone excretion is also periodically normal.

The spironolactone test is of diagnostic value (spironolactone treatment corrects hypertension and metabolic abnormalities). Topical diagnosis is not to be performed in pregnancy as it requires the use of X-ray and radionuclide techniques, while bilateral adrenal catheterization for the determination of aldosterone secretion asymmetry is a complex manipulation troublesome for the patient.

Single cases of pregnancy in patients with Conn's disease have been reported. Plasma renin activity does not increase in these patients even in pregnancy (Gordon et al. 1967). Some authors (Biglieri and Slaton 1967; Aoi et al. 1978) noted the improvement of the disease course during pregnancy, while others (Crane et al. 1964) described severe cases, complicated by preeclampsia and placental detachment, resulting in stillbith. After delivery, patients with primary aldosteronism may display a considerable blood pressure elevation and expressed hypokalemia (Aoi et al. 1978).

12.5 Pheochromocytoma

The disease is caused by a catecholamine-producing tumor of chromaffin tissue. Eighty to ninety percent of the tumors are located in adrenal medulla and 10%–20% in extramedullary chromaffin tissues (in rare cases, a bilateral tumor or combination of adrenal pheochromocytoma and extraadrenal paraganglioma is observed). The disease is relatively uncommon, but it is usually revealed in patients 20–40 years of age, i.e., in childbearing age.

There are three clinical forms of the disease: persistent, paroxysmal (with blood pressure normal outside crises), and mixed. Clinical manifestations in the persistent form are similar to those of essential hypertension. During crises (which can occur following physical exertion, and sometimes after rough pressure on the abdomen or loin, emotional stress or quite often spontaneously) the patients experience severe headache, dizziness, chest pain, palpitation, dyspnea, anxiety, fear of death, tremor, and excessive perspiration. The skin becomes pale. Nausea, vomiting, occasional pulmonary edema, convulsions, and blurring of vision are observed.

During crises, blood pressure rises up to 250/120–300/150 mmHg, and heart rhythm is disturbed. Negative T wave can be recorded on the ECG. ECG changes sometimes resemble those of myocardial infarction, which can indeed develop during severe crises, as well as cerebral hemorrhage or acute left ventricular failure accompanied by pulmonary edema. During and sometimes in between crises hyperglycemia is noted. In some cases the crisis ends with a dramatic blood pressure fall.

The diagnosis is facilitated by biochemical blood and urine examination, especially with the samples collected following the crisis. In phenochromocytoma epinephrine and norepinephrine secretion and excretion are increased, as well as the urinary level of vanillylmandelic acid. Tests employing α-adrenoblocking agents (phentolamine, phenoxybenzamine) lowering blood pressure are to be performed with caution, for fear of shock development. A histamine test, resulting in catecholamine release and blood pressure elevation, is often associated with great and even vital threat and is absolutely prohibited in pregnancy. Identification of tumor location should also be avoided in pregnancy, as it requires an X-ray examination. Pheochromocytoma manifestations in pregnant women are sometimes mistaken for preeclampsia or eclampsia in the case of convulsions.

Marked clinical manifestations of pheochromocytoma may sometimes develop or be exacerbated during pregnancy (probably partially due to the gravid uterus pressure on the tumor or to its contractions during labor), with the disease sometimes assuming a malignant course. In pregnant women with pheochromocytoma the mortality rate approaches 50% (Chesley 1978). Remission of the disease during pregnancy was also noted (Gogin et al. 1983). Schenker and Chowers (1971) summarized the data on 112 pregnancies in 89 women with pheochromocytoma. The maternal mortality rate approaches 48% (the majority of women died within 72 h after delivery) and the perinatal mortality rate was 54%. The highest death rate (58%) was noted in undiagnosed cases. The main causes of death were acute pulmonary edema and shock or, sometimes, cerebral hemorrhages, tumor hemorrhages, and fatal heart rhythm disturbances. Pregnancy in phenochromocytoma is absolutely contraindicated.

12.6 Cushing's Disease

Cushing's disease (syndrome) is caused by basophilic pituitary adenoma or some hypothalamic-pituitary disorders, resulting in increased ACTH and cortisol (as well as androgen) secretion by the pituitary gland and adrenal cortex, respectively. In recent years exogenous Cushing's syndrome has sometimes been detected, which is associated with the treatment of some diseases with high glucocorticoid doses. Cushing's disease predominates in women, mainly those of childbearing age, and though in these patients the menstrual cycle is usually disturbed, pregnancy in them is possible especially in remission and following treatment.

The patients complain of headache, fatigue, muscular weakness, sometimes pain in the bones (mainly in the spine), insomnia, and euphoria (or, on the contrary, depression). Inspection reveals typical centripetal obesity: fat depositing on the face, neck, and trunk, with arms and legs seemingly thin. The patients have red cyanotic "moon-like" faces, in some cases hirsutism. There are abdominal striae, acne, and ecchymoses on the skin.

Examination finds, as a rule, marked arterial hypertension (quite often with crises) leading to cardiac hypertrophy and precipitation of early atherosclerosis development, and, in the absence of adequate treatment, complicated by heart or renal failure or stroke. The patients often have hyperglycemia, steroid diabetes, and steroid cardiomyopathy, as well as gastrointestinal ulcers. Radiography of thoracic vertebrae reveals osteoporosis, while in roentgenography of the Turkish saddle area sometimes a pituitary adenoma is detected. Characteristic signs of the disease are: polycythemia and thrombocytosis, increased 17-hydroxycorticosteroid blood plasma level, and 17-hydroxycorticosteroid and 17-ketosteroid urinary excretion.

In Cushing's disease (syndrome) pregnancy often has an unfavorable course and outcome (early spontaneous abortion, late miscarriage and intrauterine fetal death, preeclempsia, premature labor, considerable blood loss during childbirth, stillbirth, and puerperal infection) (Grimes et al. 1973; Hadden 1982). Pregnancy in its turn has an adverse effect on the course of the disease: stable hypertension develops, which leads to heart failure, stroke, and other complications. Several cases of deaths in the puerperium have been described in women with Cushing's disease. Pregnancy in this disease is contraindicated.

12.7 Chronic Glomerulonephritis

At present the classical form of acute glomerulonephritis is a rarity. But even earlier, acute glomerulonephritis with elevated blood pressure, proteinuria, hematuria, cylindruria, and generalized edema was not a frequent pathology in the pregnant women. Sometimes it was misdiagnosed in severe preeclampsia.

Chronic glomerulonephritis is often considered the consequence of acute glomerulonephritis; however, there appears to exist a specific form of primary chronic glomerulonephritis. Streptococcal infection (acute sore throat, acute pharyngitis), cooling, and parenteral administration of heterogeneous protein seem important in the etiology of the disease. Immunological changes play an essential role in the pathogenesis of the disease. The pathogenesis of arterial hypertension in chronic glomerulonephritis remains somewhat obscure, as the disease can assume hypertensive, as well as normotensive, forms.

The hypertensive form of chronic glomerulonephritis often has no acute phase; it is not accompanied by marked changes in the urine and can, therefore, for years be mistaken for essential hypertension. This form of the disease is characterized by microhematuria and proteinuria not exceeding 1 g/liter, while the mixed form is associated with considerable proteinuria, hypoproteinemia, hyperlipidemia, lipiduria, and intermittent edema. The course of hypertension in chronic glomerulonephritis as a rule is devoid of crises, with stable diastolic pressure elevation and decrease in pulse pressure, and headache usually being less severe than in essential hypertension.

Pregnancy appears to have an adverse effect on the course of chronic glomerulonephritis, though some authors believe that the condition is aggravated only in women with a 50% reduced glomerular filtration rate, as compared with normal (Chesley 1978). However, Kincaid-Smith and Fairley (1976) have established that pregnancy aggravates the course of glomerulonephritis, for an increase in pregnancy-induced blood coagulation raises fibrin deposition in renal glomeruli. Serial biopsies have indeed revealed progressive damage of glomeruli in such patients even in a clinically normal course of pregnancy. Probably in renal diseases with even moderate renal failure, hypertension often either arises or is aggravated. In 30% of patients this is accompanied by deterioration of the renal function (Hou et al. 1985).

A number of authors have noted that chronic glomerulonephritis (as well as other chronic renal diseases) leads to a marked increase in the incidence of preeclampsia, spontaneous abortions, premature labor, and perinatal mortality rate. The maternal mortality rate during pregnancy and delivery is not usually related directly to glomerulonephritis, though in a mixed form of the disease there is a potential risk of urinary tract infection and thromboembolic complications. In some cases the patients die long after labor of severe exacerbation of glomerulonephritis, more so if manifestations of renal failure have been observed in them during pregnancy.

Pregnancy in women with the hypertensive and mixed form of glomerulonephritis is inadvisable even in adequate renal function, and when manifestations of renal failure are present it is absolutely contraindicated.

12.8 Chronic Pyelonephritis

The kidneys and urinary tract are often affected in pregnancy by an infection manifested by bacteriuria, cystitis, and acute and chronic pyelonephritis (Quilligan 1982; McGrady et al. 1985), the latter in 30%–60% of cases accompanied by arterial hypertension, sometimes assuming a malignant course. Infection is essential in the etiology of chronic pyelonephritis. The most frequent agent found in the urine is *E. coli*, which is followed by staphylococci, enterococci, *Proteus vulgaris*, and other pathogenic microorganisms. Malformations of the kidneys and urinary tract, urolithiasis, and nonspecific inflammatory diseases of the urinary bladder and urethra, as well as stricture of the urether can also play a certain role in the development of pyelonephritis. The abuse of phenacetin and phenacetin-containing analgesics contributes to the development of toxic interstitial nephritis, which can serve as the basis for chronic pyelonephritis development.

Latent chronic pyelonephritis can have only one manifestation, i.e., arterial hypertension. In this case, it is hard to differentiate it from essential hypertension if there are no definite data on pyelonephritis in the history. In the exacerbation of the disease, the patients experience discomfort, flank pain, and dysuria; sometimes fever and leukocytosis, pronounced pyuria, and mild or moderate albuminuria (not exceeding 1 g/liter) are found, and hematuria is usually insignificant except for combinations of pyelonephritis with urolithiasis.

Pregnancy promotes exacerbation of chronic pyelonephritis mainly due to urine stagnation and somewhat decreased resistance of the urinary system to infection. Chronic pyelonephritis in its turn causes a number of complications in pregnancy and can have an indirect adverse effect on the fetus. The patients often develop preeclampsia, have premature labor, and give birth to newborn with low birth weight (McGrady et al. 1985). Pregnancy is contraindicated in patients with chronic pyelonephritis accompanied by arterial hypertension and renal failure manifestations, as well as in a malignant course of hypertension and pyelonephritis of the sole kidney. In other cases, the permissibility of pregnancy and successful pyelonephritis treatment during pregnancy should be considered individually.

12.9 Collagen Diseases

Arterial hypertension in systemic lupus erythematosus (SLE), scleroderma, and periarteritis nodosa is mediated by renal involvement. As these diseases (particularly the latter two) are rare in pregnant women, their clinical pattern is not described here.

Seventy-five to ninety percent of SLE patients (90% of them female) show lupus glomerulonephritis in 25%–40% of cases accompanied by arterial hypertension. Though the data on SLE effect on pregnancy are conflicting, Chesley (1978) has summarized the data concerning 630 pregnancies, of which 64% ended in normal labor, 20% in spontaneous abortion, and 8% in stillbirth. As to the effect of pregnancy on SLE, the majority of authors believe that pregnancy is associated with exacerbation of the disease rather than with its remission, particularly in the first half of gestation and in the immediate puerperium, which in the latter case can prove fatal. This is first of all true for women with heart and renal involvement, in whom even termination of pregnancy can sometimes be fatal. Some authors believe that corticosteroid therapy in pregnancy improves the state of the patients and reduces the number of obstetric complications, while others consider it incapable of affecting the number of succesful deliveries or reducing the incidence of exacerbations. Pregnancy is contraindicated in marked SLE glomerulonephritis with elevated blood pressure. In patients with SLE showing insignificant renal disorders and transitory hypertension the decision on the permissibility of pregnancy and labor is considered individually.

Scleroderma is uncommon in pregnancy, as its clinical symptoms become usually evident only in women over 40. Some cases of pregnancies in young women with this disease have been reported. All the patients had acute blood pressure elevation and proteinuria by the end of the second trimester of pregnancy; 80% of them died. Periarteritis nodosa is also uncommon in pregnant women. Chesley (1978), summarizing the data of different authors, has reported seven such patients, who died within 4–42 days after delivery or abortion. Because of unfavorable outcomes pregnancy in scleroderma and periarteritis nodosa is believed inadmissible.

12.10 Polycystic Kidneys

Polycystic kidneys in combination with arterial hypertension is also infrequent in pregnant women, as blood pressure in this disease usually rises in patients over 40. Women under 40 with polycystic kidneys but no hypertension and renal failure usually have normal pregnancy and labor. Pregnant women with polycystic kidneys and concomitant arterial hypertension more often, as compared with obstetric patients in general, develop severe preeclampsia which can sometimes prove fatal. Hypertensive encephalopathy is also possible. In view of the above, stable hypertension in patients with polycystic kidneys is considered to be a definite contraindication of pregnancy. In labile hypertension and normal renal function pregnancy can be allowed, with the blood pressure level thoroughly monitored.

12.11 Diabetic Nephropathy

Diabetic nephropathy can occasionally develop in women of childbearing age. In 90% of cases diabetic nephropathy shown by significant proteinuria (sometimes hypercholesterolemia, rarely edema) is accompanied by arterial hypertension and retinopathy. Hypertension is evidently induced by intrarenal circulation disorders and can often assume a malignant course, especially in the presence of chronic renal failure.

Pregnancy has no marked detrimental effect on the disease (provided it is not characterized by uremia or high stable hypertension threatened with hypertensive encephalopathy). Pregnancy assumes an unfavorable course, with a high incidence of spontaneous abortions, stillbirths, and perinatal deaths. Pregnancy is contraindicated in stable arterial hypertension and/or manifestations of renal failure. In other cases the severity of diabetes mellitus should be considered.

12.12 Differential Dignosis of Arterial Hypertension

Differential diagnosis of arterial hypertension in pregnancy is often difficult, especially with no definite data on essential hypertension or secondary arterial hypertension in the history of the pregnant women. The differential diagnosis is even more difficult because X-ray and radionuclide examination, the best methods of confirming the diagnosis of most secondary hypertensions, are contraindicated in pregnancy.

The diagnosis of preeclampsia is of particular importance, for its treatment, on the one hand, helps prevent eclampsia and other complications and, on the other hand, it is a preventive measure against "posttoxemic" nephropathy, which can finally result in the development of stable arterial hypertension. Sometimes blood pressure can normalize in the first half of pregnancy in patients with essential hypertension or secondary hypertension and its increase to the usual elevated prepregnancy level is mistaken for preeclampsia (especially when it is revealed simultaneously with slight edema of the legs, which can often occur in pregnancy). On the other hand, definite signs of preeclampsia cannot in some cases exclude the presence of preexisting essential hypertension or secondary hypertension (Eliseev 1982).

In doubtful cases, diagnosis of essential hypertension can be facilitated by familial history of hypertension, early (prior to week 20 of gestation) onset of hypertension, lack of proteinuria and edema, presence of characteristic changes of the eyegrounds, clinical and electrocardiographic findings of left ventricular hypertrophy, as well as normal uric acid clearance. These findings should be taken into consideration mainly in the differential diagnosis of preeclampsia, as some of them can also be found in secondary hypertensions (Eliseev 1979).

Preeclampsia usually develops after the 20th week of gestation (except for cases of trophoblastic disease, in which this syndrome can be found earlier) and is more frequent in primigravidas. Increased serum level of uric and retinal artery angiospasm are typical features of preeclampsia (Finnerty 1977). In preeclampsia blood pressure elevation is too short term for left ventricular hypertrophy to develop. Eclampsia episodes should be differentiated from epileptic fits and eclamptic coma from diabetic and uremic coma.

Renovascular hypertension diagnosis in pregnancy can be based only on clinical data. In the majority of cases, hypertension is stable, is free of crises, and responds poorly to active antihypertensive therapy; however, sometimes hypertension is malignant, diastolic pressure is predominantly elevated, and in the first half of pregnancy abdominal bruit is auscultated above the area of origin of the renal arteries. No albuminuria and alterations of urinary sediment are usually observed. In patients with Takayasu's disease pulsation in one or both radial arteries is either absent or attenuated.

Diagnosis of Conn's disease in the presence of high hypertension, attacks of hypokalemia-mediated pronounced muscular weakness, paresthesias, polydipsia, polyuria, aldosteronuria, hypokalemia, and hyporeninemia is quite easy. The diagnosis is facilitated by the spironolactone test. It should be recognized that Conn's disease has an intermittent course and its symptoms can be weakly expressed (particularly in summer and autumn when a lot of potassium-containing vegetable food is consumed).

Differential diagnosis of pheochromocytoma can prove difficult in both the presence and absence of crises. Detection of hyperglycemia and glucosuria, poorly responding to insulin injections, can be of some value. The phentolamine test can be helpful.

Diagnosis of Cushing's disease (syndrome) is usually easy due to typical clinical manifestations. The diagnosis can be verified by laboratory tests (elevation of 17-hydroxycorticosteroid blood plasma level, and increased 17-hydroxycorticosteroid and 17-ketosteroid urinary excretion).

The urinary syndrome being weakly expressed, the hypertensive form of chronic glomerulonephritis is to be differentiated from essential hypertension, the hypertensive form of chronic pyelonephritis, renovascular hypertension, and other forms of arterial hypertension, characterized by slight urinary changes. It should be recognized that in essential hypertension the urinary syndrome develops years after the onset of hypertension, while in chronic glomerulonephritis it either precedes hypertension or their onsets are simultaneous. Glomerulonephritis almost never gives hypertensive crises, while a reduced glomerular filtration rate is observed along with a moderate decrease of renal blood flow. In essential hypertension, on the contrary, renal blood flow is considerably diminished, the glomerular filtration rate remaining normal for a long period (Ratner 1974). Differentiation from chronic pyelonephritis may be facilitated by urinary sediment examination (erythrocytes prevail in glomerulonephritis; leukocytes prevail in pyelonephritis). In renovascular hypertension there may be no changes in the urinary sediment, with blood pressure being, as a rule, extremely stable.

The history of the acute phase of the disease or its exacerbations with concomitant flank pain, dysuria, pyuria, and sometimes fever, and in some cases information on renal colic episodes and calculi appearance in the urine as well as on phenacetin abuse, can prove very helpful for the diagnosis of chronic pyelonephritis or analgesic nephritis, respectively. Great attention is attached to characteristic changes in the urinary sediment and expressed bacteriuria, as well as to a reduction of renal tubular reabsorption (polyuria and hypostenuria) and diminution of maximal tubular paraaminohippuric acid secretion (with the latter changes being commonly typical of bilateral pyelonephritis).

Diagnosis of SLE, scleroderma, periarteritis nodosa, and diabetes mellitus is quite easy in the presence of their definite clinical manifestations. Primary diagnosis of polycystic kidneys is impossible in pregnancy, for it requires findings of roentgenourological studies.

In many unclear cases of arterial hypertension diagnosis is facilitated by biopsy of the kidneys. But, in pregnancy, this diagnostic procedure is to be avoided in the majority of cases as there is the risk (however minimal) of postpuncture bleeding. Renal biopsy in the postpartal period is obligatory if the woman retains so-called postnephropathic (posttoxemic) hypertension, and the diagnosis remains unclear. The most frequent causes of such hypertension are preexisting latent chronic glomerulonephritis and essential hypertension (Kozdoba 1970).

12.13 Management of Patients with Arterial Hypertension

Pregnant women with arterial hypertension (or proteinuria even in normal BP) should be admitted into special high-risk pregnancy units of a maternity hospital, where the diagnosis is verified, the possibility of safe pregnancy is considered, and an adequate therapy is prescribed. Pregnant women with high arterial hypertension should be kept in bed (the lateral position is preferable) and should receive antihypertensive drugs, with limited sodium intake. Sodium restriction in preeclampsia is not always indisputable: in preeclampsia there is relative hypovolemia and sometimes (as in some patients with malignant hypertension) a salt-free diet and diuretics can produce an even more marked reduction in plasma volume accompanied by mounting placental ischemia, renal hemodynamic disturbances (Foidart and Rorive 1977), and deterioration of maternal and fetal condition. Pregnant women with arterial hypertension are admitted into a maternity hospital 2–3 weeks before term.

Pregnant women with arterial hypertension should be examined in outpatient clinics (urine analyses obligatory) every 2 weeks and, after the 30th week, every week, and should be hospitalized in case their blood pressure rises, or if they have hypertensive crises or manifestations of preeclampsia.

As in patients with heart disease, in hypertensive pregnant women it is essential to regulate a proper work-rest regimen, do away with detrimental occupational factors, calm the patient down with sedative drugs, and ensure a sound 8- to 10-h sleep (1–2 h may be, if possible, spent as an afternoon nap). Antihypertensive therapy is performed with a diastolic pressure level exceeding 90 mmHg; blood pressure should be measured with the patient in the sitting position as there may be a 10- to 15-mmHg blood pressure fall in supine pregnant women (Gallery 1980). In mild hypertension (diastolic BP <95 mmHg) medical therapy is not always necessary: rest, relaxation, mild physical exercise, restricted salt, and a calorie-controlled diet might suffice. In moderate hypertension the above measures are combined with drug therapy. The therapy is aimed at the prevention of both hypertension complications and preeclampsia-eclampsia.

When choosing appropriate antihypertensive drugs and adjusting their doses it is necessary to bear in mind that abrupt blood pressure fall impairs uteroplacental circulation and that rather many of the drugs may affect the fetus. Thiazide and some other diuretics (often in combination with antihypertensive drugs) have long been used, as they have a moderate antihypertensive and, in the case of fluid retention, diuretic effect. Thiazide diuretics cross the placenta with no reported teratogenic effect on the fetus although occasional thrombocytopenia (Sullivan 1974), hypokalemia, and hyponatremia (Kunz and Schreiner 1982) were noted in the newborn.

In their review Collins et al. (1985) report that at least 11 randomized studies on the use of diuretics for the prevention of preeclampsia and its sequelae have been performed over a 20-year period. Nine of them included about 7000 pregnant women.

The success was undoubted even if edema was not included in the diagnostic criteria. The incidence of stillbirths declined by one-third; however, postnatal survival was but slightly affected. However, some authors are sceptical as to the use of diuretics in hypertensive pregnant women as their antihypertensive effect is modest, whereas there is the risk of an undesirable reduction in blood volume and uteroplacental circulation, as well as the onset of maternal hypokalemia (Murnaghan 1982; Lubbe 1984; etc.).

Hydrochlorothiazide is usually given daily in week courses with 1-week intervals, on in long-term courses every other day. The dose is individually adjusted and accounts for 25–100 mg/day. Mean doses of other saluretics (chlorthalidone, clopamide) are also used. To avoid hypokalemia in long-term treatment with saluretics a high potassium diet is recommended and oral potassium preparations, as well as potassium-sparing drugs (spironolactone, triamterene, amiloride), are given.

Oral antihypertensive therapy with furosemide and etacrinic acid does not seem expedient during pregnancy. Their parenteral injection is useful in hypertensive crises and pulmonary edema. Furosemide is to be used when diuretics are indicated in pregnant women with renal failure. The use of captopril, an inhibitor of angiotensin-converting enzyme, in pregnant women with severe hypertension is open to debate. There have been reports on the teratogenic effect of the drug (Duminy and Burger 1981), a high percentage of stillbirths, and a case of early perinatal death (Broughton-Pupkin et al. 1982). However, Mochizuki et al. (1986) have successfully used captopril in combination with other antihypertensive agents in late pregnancy in patients with severe hypertension refractory to other medication. No side effects have been observed.

Long-term reserpine application in doses exceeding 0.5 mg/day is inadvisable in pregnant women. And as reserpine crosses the placenta and enters breast milk to cause enhanced secretion in airways, nasal mucosa congestion, cyanosis, and anorexia in the newborn, it should not be administered prior to and following labor. As reserpine is in some cases capable of causing maternal depression, it is better to avoid its use in gestation (Lubbe 1984).

Methyldopa at a dose of 0.5–2 g/day is rather frequently used in pregnancy. As the drug causes fluid retention, it should be used in combination with low doses of diuretics. Clonidine is given orally at a dose of 0.15–1.2 mg/day, and injected intravenously or intramuscularly during hypertensive crises at a dose of 0.15–0.3 mg (the drug should be slowly infused intravenously in 10–20 ml of normal saline solution). Sudden cessation of treatment with this drug can give rise to a hypertensive crisis.

Guanethidine, which induces severe orthostatic hypotension, is used in pregnancy at a dose of 12.5–50 mg/day only if other antihypertensive drugs are ineffective. Caution should be exercised when using guanethidine in patients with reduced renal function, as it decreases renal blood flow and glomerular filtration rate. If there is to be surgical intervention, administration of guanethidine should be stopped 1 week before the operation. Guanethidine should be avoided, if possible, as orthostatic hypotension has a detrimental effect on uteroplacental perfusion. The above three drugs do not have an unfavorable effect on the fetus.

Diazoxide has a marked antihypertensive effect in pregnant women, but its application can cause sodium and water retention in the mother, as well as hypoxia, hyperglycemia, hyperbilirubinemia, and thrombocytopenia in the fetus; therefore, its long-term administration should be avoided. Intravenous infusion of 150–300 mg diazoxide effectively lowers elevated blood pressure during hypertensive crises in pregnancy; since there is the risk of potential abrupt BP lowering, 150 mg of the drug should be slowly infused first, and then, if necessary, 60 mg of the drug can be infused twice. Hydralazine is also infused intravenously; in hypertensive crises the drug dose is individually adjusted, beginning with 20 mg; the infusion is continued at a rate of 2–20 mg/h under BP monitoring every 5–10 min and then every 15–30 min (Lubbe 1984). In the treatment course, hydralazine is given orally at a dose of 40–300 mg/day. In cases of emergency intravenous injections of ganglioblockers (hexametonium-bromide, etc.) are possible. Ganglioblockers are inappropriate for a course of antihypertensive treatment, as along with numerous side effects in the mother they also cause meconium ileus and urine bladder atony in the newborn.

There is still no full agreement on the use of beta-blockers in pregnant women with hypertension. Dubois and Petitcolas (1977), Eliahou et al. (1978), Gallery (1980), and some other authors are for the use of beta-blockers in these cases. Hawkins (1976), Lieberman et al. (1978), and others reported the adverse effect of beta-blockers on the fetus, especially in placental blood flow insufficiency. In recent years convincing data have appeared on the expediency of using beta-blockers, alfa-blockers, and their combinations in hypertensive pregnant patients. Their advantages are gradual onset of action, the absence of a negative effect on the plasma volume, and the lack of drug-induced postural hypotension. A number of studies have shown that pindolol at a dose of 10–30 mg/day is effective in reducing systolic and diastolic blood pressure and increasing uteroplacental circulation, and has no side effects in the mother and fetus, the mean birth weight being higher than in the control group (Ingemarsson et al. 1984; Kahhale et al. 1984; Lunnell et al. 1984; Tuimala and Hartikainen-Sorri 1984). The incidence of premature labor and low birth weight of neonates was not higher than the expected rates for a population of this nature (Sukerman-Voldman 1982). Along with pindolol; acebutolol, atenolol (Dubois et al 1983; Rubin et al. 1983, 1984) and other beta-blockers (Lindberg and Sandström 1981) were effectively used. However, in recent years it has also sometimes been believed that beta-blockers in hypertensive pregnant patients should be used with caution, while their combined use with other antihypertensive drugs, which makes it possible to diminish the drug doses and reduce the likelihood of side effects, is considered promising (Ticconi et al. 1985).

In hypertensive pregnant women combined alpha- and beta-blockade seems advisable. Thus, according to some authors, alpha- and beta-blocker labetalol (Garden et al. 1982) and the combination of the alpha-blocker prazosin with one of the beta-blockers oxprenolol, pindolol, or atenolol (Lubbe 1984) are extremely effective. Monotherapy with prazosin at a dose of 6–30 mg/day is also effective in hypertensive pregnant women (Stanaszek et al. 1983; Wicker and Dallachio 1984).

There are data on successful sublingual administration of 5–20 mg calcium antagonist nifedipine in pregnant women with severe hypertension and hypertensive crises including those refractory to routine antihypertensive drugs (Walters and Redman 1982; Papi et al. 1985). The successful use of intravenous prostaglandin I_2 infusion in pregnant women with severe hypertension has been reported (Belch et al. 1985) as well as preeclampsia control by the administration of the serotonin receptor antagonist ketanserin (Weiner et al. 1984).

It should be recognized that many antihypertensive agents contribute to sodium and water retention and that saluretics cause marked sodium (and potassium) urinary loss. Therefore, the combination of reduced drug doses not only potentiates their antihypertensive action, but also, to some extent, attenuates their adverse effects (Eliseev 1982).

In preeclampsia-eclampsia, antihypertensive agents are not always sufficiently effective; therefore, intramuscular injection of magnesium sulfate (2.5–10 g) and chlorpromazine (100–150 mg) prove to be useful, with the drugs infused intravenously in eclampsia (slow 20-min infusions of 4 g magnesium sulfate in 100 ml dextrose solution are, if necessary, followed by intravenous maintenance infusions; intravenous infusions of 25–50 mg chlorpromazine are possible; pethidine is also applied). In eclampsia use is also made of short-acting barbiturates, diazepam first injected intramuscularly (10 mg) and then drip infused (40 mg in 500 ml 5% glucose), diazoxide (300 mg intravenously), droperidol, and halothane.

It is recommended to terminate pregnancy within 24–48 h after the cessation of eclampsia convulsions (Sokolow and McIlroy 1981). If refractory preeclampsia persists for several days, pregnancy should be terminated either by labor induction (near term) or by cesarean section (Perloff 1984).

A proper work-rest regimen, a well-balanced low-salt diet, administration of low diuretic doses at the initial stage or in preeclampsia (when the plasma volume is augmented and not reduced), and antihypertensive drugs in blood pressure elevation — all these contribute to the prevention of preeclampsia-eclampsia. Diastolic blood pressure should be maintained at a level not exceeding 90 mmHg and diuresis should be not less than 1.5 liter/day. Reports have appeared on the possibility of preventing pregnancy-induced hypertension and preeclampsia in angiotensin-sensitive primigravidas by small doses (60 mg/day) of aspirin (Wallenburg 1986). Women who have had severe preeclampsia or eclampsia should be advised to resort to careful contraception or probably even sterilization.

Some secondary hypertensions also require, in addition to antihypertensive therapy, etiological and pathogenetic treatment.

As localization of renal artery occlusions in renovascular hypertension and tumor locations in Conn's disease and pheochromocytoma are mostly unknown in pregnant women, surgery in these diseases is not as a rule performed during pregnancy. In stable high hypertension termination of pregnancy is advisable, and surgery following thorough examination of such patients is recommended. In Conn's disease spironolactone therapy (200–400 mg/day) may prove effective. Successful therapy with alpha-blockers, namely phenoxybenzamine, is possible in pheochromocytoma. There is an opinion that the tumor should be, if possible, excised in the first trimester of pregnancy, while in the second and third trimesters adequate therapy with alpha-blockers is necessary until term; then cesarean section is performed, which is followed by surgical removal of the tumor (Stenstrom and Swolin 1985). The use of metyrapone made it possible to reduce cortisol secretion during pregnancy in patients with Cushing's syndrome (Gormley et al. 1982).

Corticosteroids, in large doses, cytostatic and aminochinoline drugs, indomethacin, and immunosuppressors currently used for the treatment of chronic glomerulonephritis are contraindicated in pregnancy due to their damaging effect on the fetus. The only possible agent seems to be heparin injected at a dose of 20000 units per day for 20–40 days.

Antibacterial agents are very important for the treatment of chronic pyelonephritis and its exacerbations in particular; however, they should be used in pregnancy with regard to their possible effect on the fetus. In the first trimester of pregnancy intramuscular injections of natural and semisynthetic penicillins in high doses (penicillin, 8000000–10000000 units/day; ampicillin, 2 g/day; carbenicillin, 4 g/day) for 8 to 10 days would suffice (Shekhtman 1980). In the second and third trimesters of pregnancy other antibiotics can be used (except for tetracylcine, chloramphenicol, and aminoglycosides) in conventional doses, as well as other antibacterial drugs. Sulfacarbamidum (its use should be avoided in the antepartal period) in exacerbations of the disease is given at a dose of 5–6 g/day on the 1st day of treatment and then 3–4 g/day, with the dose in the latent course of the disease accounting for 2–3 g/day. Nitrofurantoin is prescribed at a dose of 0.4 g/day for 5 days and 0.3 g/day for 10 days. Acidum nalidixicum is used at a dose of 6 g/day for 5 days and 2 g/day for another 10-day period. Nitroxoline is given at a dose of 100 mg four to six times/day for 2 weeks. The drug choice should be based on microbial sensitivity tests in urine culture and individual drug tolerance. Treating pyelonephritis in the puerpera, one should be aware of the possible penetration of some drugs (aminoglycosides and sulfonamides) into breast milk. Sometimes for urine drainage recovery, ureter catheterization is used. In severe cases, surgery (kidney decapsulation, nephrostomy) and detoxication therapy are indicated.

In systemic lupus erythematosus, treatment with azathioprine, dipyridamole, heparin, and prednisolone is performed (Kincaid-Smith 1975; Hayslett and Lynn 1980). Corticosteroids are recommended in the first half of pregnancy and especially in the early puerperium (Chesley 1978). In diabetic nephropathy treatment of diabetes mellitus is performed.

Delivery in arterial hypertension should be vaginal and performed under analgesia (as in cardiac patients). Prior to labor, it is advisable to normalize or reduce blood pressure. If this cannot be achieved, labor efforts should be avoided by using outlet forceps delivery. Bearing in mind possible blood loss during labor and other hypotensive effects, antihypertensive drugs in mild and moderate hypertension may be discontinued or their doses may be reduced 2–3 days before term. Sometimes cesarean section is indicated (in cerebral blood flow disorders, severe changes of the eyegrounds, severe preeclampsia, or obstetric pathology).

No data concerning special trials on the effects of antihypertensive drugs on breast-fed infants have been reported. Only case reports or data based on studies in small groups of lactating women have been published. According to a brief review (White 1984), although practically all antihypertensive agents penetrate into the breast milk (some of them in concentrations higher than in maternal plasma), no adverse effects on the babies were noted, except for reserpine, which caused significant nasal congestion in the newborn. It is important to bear in mind that thiazide diuretics can suppress lactation; therefore their use as antihypertensive agents should be avoided in lactating women.

Women whose blood pressure was elevated in pregnancy (even if it normalized after delivery) should be carefully followed up after childbirth by a cardiologist or internist.

Irrespective of the origin of hypertension in high, stable blood pressure elevation with severe changes of the eyegrounds, in heart failure, coronary insufficiency, or renal failure, or in impaired cerebral circulation threatening with cerebral hemorrhage, termination of pregnancy is vitally important. Pregnancy is terminated early by therapeutic abortion and later by cesarean section, preferably following blood pressure reduction to an almost normal level.

13 Arterial Hypotension and Pregnancy

Arterial hypotension should not be considered a specific nosological form. In some healthy women (namely, in sportswomen) it can be their peculiar normal BP level; in others it is associated with disturbances of neurohumoral mechanisms regulating circulation and is a manifestation of so-called neurocirculatory hypotensive dystonia (essential or idiopathic hypotension), while in another group of patients, as in those with symptomatic hypertension, it is a symptom of some particular disease (adrenal insufficiency, diabetic neuropathy, anemia, infectious disease, hypothyroidism, etc.). BP fall usually occurs on assuming an upright posture (orthostatic hypotension).

The etiology and pathogenesis of orthostatic hypotension so far are unclear despite numerous studies and hypotheses; consequently there is no point in criticizing some and praising others. In pregnancy, along with other reasons, in patients with insufficient adaptation of BP-regulating apparatus, physiological increase of vascular bed capacity, blood retention in the veins of lower extremities, and hormonal shifts can all contribute to BP lowering.

It has been established that pregnant women with primary arterial hypotension have deteriorated cerebral hemodynamics and some disturbances of the brain cortex, hypothalamus, and reticular formation functions: acetylcholine and histamine blood levels are often increased; while adrenaline, noradrenaline, serotonin, and oxycorticosteroid blood levels are diminished (Schatz 1980; Rakut 1981).

Blood pressure below 100/60 mmHg is rather often detected in young women (arterial hypotension predominates in women), including pregnant ones, and can be asymptomatic. In some such women, as pregnancy advances, BP increases, reaching a physiologically normal level, or in rare cases exceeding it. It should be noted that in nonpregnant women there are cases of orthostatic hypotension transforming into essential hypertension, but abnormal blood pressure elevation in pregnant women suffering from hypotension is commonly a sign of superimposed preeclampsia. The incidence of arterial hypotension in pregnant women is rather high: according to Vogler (1968), it is about 30%, according to Bergman (1983), it is 10.9%, 70.8% of all the cases being practically asymptomatic. In primigravidas arterial hypotension is observed more often; it usually develops in the 13th–14th weeks of gestation and is revealed mostly in the 17th–24th weeks, while near term it is established in 7.7% of women (Bergman 1983).

The patients often complain of profound weakness, emotional unrest, reduced working capacity, dizziness (sometimes also headache), unpleasant sensations in the heart area (sometimes stabbing chest pain), sweating, cold hands and feet, and paresthesias. The symptoms are sometimes aggravated with weather changes. Some patients on assuming an upright posture experience dizziness, blurred vision, tinnitus, shortness of breath, sweating, nausea (seldom vomiting), and, occasionally, syncope. History data sometimes reveal long-term emotional strain, psychic trauma, intensive mental work, and viral infections.

On inspection, patients with arterial hypotension demonstrate asthenic body constitution, skin pallor, mild acrocyanosis, hyperhydrosis (most marked in armpit areas), reduced skin temperature in the hands and feet, and red dermographism. The heart size is, as a rule, normal (occasionally so-called tear-drop heart is radiographically revealed). Sometimes faint systolic murmur over the heart apex is audible. In marked hypotension heart sounds can be somewhat muffled. Bradycardia is frequent; rather pronounced respiratory arrhythmia and rare premature beats can sometimes be revealed. The pulse is labile, especially in emotional and physical strain, BP is below 100/60 mmHg, and pulse pressure is often decreased. Twenty-four-hour monitoring (Gembitsky 1982) reveals marked BP lability or sometimes even episodes of its elevation above the normal level. The ECG voltage is sometimes reduced. Impedance plethysmographic findings are those of reduced tone and elasticity both in major and minor peripheral vessels and opposite shifts in central vessels, while electroencephalographically pathological brain biopotentials are recorded (Bergman 1983). Peripheral vascular resistance is decreased, cardiac output can be somewhat elevated, and circulation time is increased.

In patients with orthostatic hypotension, assumption of the upright posture or prolonged standing are followed not only by subjective disorders but also by a dramatic BP fall, frequently heart rate decrease and sometimes tachycardia. These disorders promptly disappear with the patient in the recumbent position. In rare cases, patients with arterial hypotension may have hypotensive crises, sometimes accompanied by signs of cerebral blood flow disturbances (Kulago 1974). The possible effect of occupational factors on the development of secondary hypotension should be taken into consideration (low doses of ionizing radiation, electromagnetic radiation, noise, vibration, chronic mercury, nitrobenzene, tetraethyllead and trinitrotoluene intoxication, etc.).

Pregnant women with arterial hypotension have a twice higher incidence of complications during labor than normotensive women; they show more often disturbed attachment and separation of the placenta and postpartal bleedings, malformations in offspring of such women being 2.5 times more frequent than in normotensive women (Rimbach and Heiligstein 1967). Women with arterial hypotension more often than normotensive women have premature labor, premature membrane rupture, weak expulsive efforts, blood loss during labor and in the puerperium, intrauterine fetal hypoxia, asphyxia of neonates, stillbirths, and early perinatal death (Bekker 1975; Rakut 1981; Bergman 1983); there is an increased threat of spontaneous abortion and preeclampsia (Legostaev and Drozdov 1978). Pregnant patients with arterial hypotension reveal significant histological, histochemical, and ultrastructural changes of the placenta. Therefore, it seems possible that the majority of the above obstetric complications are associated with disturbed uteroplacental and fetoplacental circulation, and, in large part, can be prevented or removed by timely and effective therapy.

Nonpharmacological measures are essential in the treatment of arterial hypotension: adequate work-rest regimen, elimination of harmful occupational factors, physical and psychoemotional strain, a sufficient (not less than 8–9 h) night's sleep (preferably with the head of the bed elevated to 5°–20°), gradual transition from the recumbent to the sitting posture and from the sitting to the standing posture after sleep, swimming (exit from the water must be gradual), and massage and isotonic physical exercise, such as walking. In the morning a cup (not more) of strong coffee or tea seems useful. In mild cases, usual doses of ginseng root and similar vegetable stimulators of the autonomic nervous system will suffice. It should be recognized that there is an individual tolerance both to the above preparations and to the most potent drugs used in the treatment of arterial hypotension. Therefore, the most effective drug or combination of drugs should be selected. Etilefrin (5 mg two to three times/day) for 3–4 weeks, if necessary, can be used repeatedly at any time during pregnancy and preventively for 2 weeks before childbirth (Bergman 1976). In marked hypotension, 1 ml of a 1% etilefrine solution is injected subcutaneously or intramuscularly during labor, and if repeated injections are required they are performed at 2- to 3-h intervals. A beta-sympathomimetic isoprenaline (5 mg sublingually three times a day) can be used (Voronin 1986). As orthostatic arterial hypotension is almost always accompanied by venous insufficiency associated with blood deposition in the leg veins, Goeschen et al. (1985) have successfully used dihydroergotamine, a drug possessing venotonic properties (2.5 mg twice a day for 10 days) in pregnant women. The drugs of choice are probably caffeine and nicethamide. Ephedrine and phenylephedrine (0.025 g and 0.01 g two to three times/day, respectively) are commonly used in combination with other drugs. In the second half of pregnancy desoxycorticosterone acetate (1 ml of 0.5% solution) is administered intramuscularly or 10 mg/day of prednisolone is administered in a short-term oral course (it is advisable to increase potassium intake in this period). According to Grünberger et al. (1978), children born to mothers treated in this manner had no symptoms of hypotrophy and had a considerably higher birth weight in comparison with children from the control group (whose hypotensive mothers received no corticosteroids). The drug of choice is 9-alpha-fludrocortisone; it is started at 0.1–0.2 mg daily and can be titrated to 2.0 mg daily (Onrot et al. 1986). However, it must be acknowledged that fluoridized corticosteroids are teratogenic (Kunz and Schreiner 1982) and, therefore, the drugs are not recommended in the first half of pregnancy.

In recent years successful attempts at arterial hypotension treatment with levodopa per se or in combination with corticosteroids (Schatz 1980) and metoclopramide (dopaminergic receptor antagonist) (Kuchel et al. 1980) were made. However, the use of the former drug in pregnancy has not been investigated, while the latter has been successfully used in pregnancy against vomiting. There is a report on the efficacy and safety of mephentermine in pregnant women suffering from arterial hypotension (Lauckner et al. 1978). Systolic and diastolic blood pressure in response to this drug considerably rises due to cardiac output increase, while heart rate and systemic peripheral resistance remain practically unchanged. Such a hemodynamic situation is favorable for uteroplacental circulation (the blood flow is increased).

Retrosternal pain occurring sometimes in patients with severe orthostatic hypotension is mediated by coronary blood flow insufficiency. And nitroglycerin, having a venodilating effect and thus aggravating hypotension, can strengthen the pain. The pain is relieved on assuming a recumbent posture or following administration of vasopressor drugs, e.g., phenylephrine.

Uteroplacental circulation increase enhances placental perfusion; therefore any therapy contributing to BP normalization improves fetal blood supply and nutrition. Thus, treatment of arterial hypotension should be performed in all pregnant women whose BP level is below 105/60 mmHg, even if they are asymptomatic (Eliseev 1982).

A high-protein diet with relatively liberal salt intake, coffee, and tea consumption, and vitamin B_1, B_6, B_{12}, and ascorbic acid administration are of additional value in the treatment of arterial hypotension. Oxygen therapy and hyperbaric oxygenation have a favorable effect (Voronin et al. 1986), and elastic stockings are advisable. There are reports on successful laser irradiation on biologically active points in pregnant women with hypotension (Didia et al. 1983). Some authors recommend anabolic steroids (Pokalev 1974), monoamine oxidase inhibitors in combination with tyramine-containing food products (Diamond et al. 1970), and indomethacin (Kochar and Itzkovitz 1978). However, they do not seem advisable in pregnancy due to their possible unfavorable effect on the fetus. To improve uteroplacental circulation pentoxyphilline (100 mg, three times/day) can be used, beginning with the second trimester of pregnancy (Voronin et al. 1986).

In symptomatic arterial hypotension the underlying disease causing it should be treated, bearing in mind potential drug effects on the fetus.

Adequate, individually adjusted, timely therapy makes it possible not only to remove symptoms caused by arterial hypotension, but also to prevent the development of numerous complications during pregnancy and labor.

Arterial hypotension in the puerperium is also a problem, as it delays rehabilitation of the mother and renders difficult her care of the newborn. The use of some drugs received in the antepartal period is inadvisable in nursing mothers. This, for instance, concerns corticosteroids. There are reports on a successful use of postsynaptic receptor activator dimetophrine (200 mg three times/day) in postpartal hypotension. Systolic and diastolic pressure levels promptly normalized, subjective disorders were removed, and no side effects were noted either in the mother or in nursed babies (Marsoni 1985). Termination of pregnancy in arterial hypotension in the absence of other indications is not required.

14 Vascular Diseases and Pregnancy

14.1 Diseases of the Aorta and Arteries

There are data that the release of high amounts of female sex hormones during pregnancy (namely, yellow body hormones) mediate certain changes in the vascular wall structure and aggravate the course of vascular diseases, thereby increasing the mortality rate from them.

The incidence of aortic dissection and rupture of the aortic and spleen artery aneurysm is higher in pregnant than in nonpregnant women of the corresponding age group (Quilligan 1982). Ten to twenty percent of all maternal deaths are caused by vascular catastrophies, including 2%–5% of deaths by intracranial hemorrhages (Danforth 1982). Pregnant women infrequently reveal telangiectasia and arteriovenous fistulas in the extremities. A higher incidence of intracranial and carotid artery occlusion in preexisting diseases is observed during pregnancy and after labor.

14.1.1 Dissecting Aortic Aneurysm

Pregnancy which is always accompanied by BV increase and sometimes by BP elevation and progressing degenerative process in the aortic media is considered one of the causes of the dissection of the aorta (Roberts 1981). Aortic dissection usually develops in the antepartal period (predominantly in the third trimester of gestation) and is much less frequent during labor or in the early puerperium. BP elevation that occurs prior to aortic dissection is detected in about 50% of cases. The risk of aortic dissection is rather high in women with Marfan's syndrome, coarctation of the aorta, and congenital bicuspid aortic valve (Gore and Seiwert 1952; Murdoch et al. 1972). In Marfan's syndrome there is a congenital cystous degeneration of the aortic media, with the pathological process possibly causing aortic root dilation and aortic wall thinning. According to data in the literature, pregnancy in women with Marfan's syndrome is fatal in 10%–40% of cases. Therefore, a regular echocardiographic control over the state of the aortic root is obligatory (Lind and Van Papendrecht 1984), which helps to detect advancing dilation of the aortic root and thus a tendency toward its rupture. Pregnancy is contraindicated in patients with marked changes of the aortic root.

Coarctation of the aorta may be accompanied not only by its dissection but also by its rupture (Nesbitt and Abdul-Karim 1982). The presence of coarctation of the aorta can in certain circumstances be an indication for the termination of pregnancy, its surgical correction during pregnancy, and, finally, cesarean section. It should be recognized that the previous correction of the defect does not guarantee the patient will not have complications during subsequent pregnancies. Aortic dissection proximal to the coarctation area (Murnaghan 1982) and even rupture of the graft (Davis and Leider 1977) are possible.

In acute dissection of the chest aorta the patients experience strong retrosternal or back pain, often accompanied by a collapse. This clinical picture is sometimes considered a manifestation of myocardial infarction. The pain in dissection of the abdominal part of the aorta sometimes resembles renal colic. The pain can irradiate up to the small pelvis in distal dissection and can be at times attenuated. Pulse asymmetry in the arms or legs with disturbed circulation in the extremities often occurs. In gradual aortic dissection, heart failure can develop, while the compression of renal artery ostia gives rise to uremia. In both cases the mortality rate is very high.

The electrocardiographic findings make it possible to rule out myocardial infarction, while echocardiography may reveal signs of aortic dissection. Radiographic findings reveal a considerable broadening of the aortic shadow.

Patients with aortic dissection require bed rest, effective analgesia, administration of the drugs reducing myocardial contractility (beta-blockers), and antihypertensive therapy in the case of BP elevation. Upon relieving the pain attack and BP normalization, the pregnant woman should be transported to a cardiosurgical hospital, where surgery is considered. Surgery is usually followed by the termination of pregnancy. In the absence of indications for urgent interventions on the aorta, pregnancy should be terminated for fear of further progession of the aortic dissection, with the patient referred to a surgical clinic for surgical treatment.

14.1.2 Arterial Aneurysms

Arterial aneurysm, predominating in females, poses a serious threat to the life of pregnant women. The mortality rate in patients with aneurysm ruptures can exceed 75%. In the majority of cases, spleen (their rupture is most frequent between the 7th and 9th months of pregnancy), cerebral, renal, and iliac artery aneurysms are detected. Coronary artery aneurysm is less frequent (however, its rupture is almost always fatal). The factor promoting aneurysm rupture is mainly arterial hypertension and, less frequently, strain during labor (Fujita et al. 1978; Miniely et al. 1979). Timely diagnosis and surgical correction of an aneurysm (sometimes even performed during pregnancy) can contribute to the decrease in maternal mortality. In the presence of great artery aneurysm, pregnancy is contraindicated.

14.1.3 Takayasu's Disease

Takayasu's (pulseless) disease is chronic inflammatory arteriopathy of unknown etiology, affecting the aorta and its main branches (rather often also the pulmonary artery). The disease is complicated by secondary hypertension, aortic regurgitation, ischemic retinopathy, and also aortic and arterial aneurysms. The incidence of the disease is eight to nine times higher in females than in males. Takayasu's syndrome is most frequently detected by the loss of radial pulse on one or both arms as well as by attenuation (or even loss) of carotid pulse. The latter case is frequently characterized by syncope.

Blood pressure should be measured on the legs, as it may be false normal on the arms. Pregnancy, contrary to widespread opinion, probably has no obvious negative effect on the course of the disease. However, according to summarized data, various cardiovascular complications during pregnancy, labor, and puerperium are observed in 61.4% of cases, including 4.8% of deaths from brain hemorrages during labor (Ishikawa and Matsuura 1982). The most frequent complications of pregnancy are not rupture of aneurysm but heart failure, a rise of an already elevated blood pressure, and a superimposed preeclampsia. Cerebral hemorrhage can be accompanied by convulsions, as in the case of eclampsia. Low or moderate corticosteroid doses can be given if an active inflammatory process is retained or is exacerbated during pregnancy. Preventive therapy with antibiotics against the onset of bacterial endocarditis and septicemia is obligatory in all these patients during labor and in the puerperium. While performing antihypertensive therapy, it should be recognized that a drop in blood pressure in patients with carotid artery lesions can lead to syncope. During labor it seems expedient to use outlet forceps or a vacuum extractor. Cesarean section is indicated in severe narrowing of the aortic arch, dramatic BP elevation in the first stage of labor, preeclampsia, and severe retinopathy. If necessary, anticoagulants are administered (Ishikawa and Matsuura 1982).

14.2 Diseases of the Veins

14.2.1 Varicose Veins

Varicose changes in the veins of the lower extremities are detected, according to different authors, in 20%–50% of pregnant women. They are sometimes combined with varicosities in the pelvic veins, veins of the hemorrhoidal plexus, pudendal veins, and sometimes breast veins. Hormonal influence may, to a great extent, be a precipitating factor; the disease predominates in females. The disease is frequently first seen during pregnancy due to reduced tone of venous wall smooth muscles induced by excessive levels of female sexual hormones (Wenner 1979), and also due to the rise in intraperitoneal and venous pressure. Hereditary and some occupational factors (e.g., prolonged standing disturbs venous outflow) play a certain role in the development of the disease. Morphological and functional changes of the venous wall and valves promote a rise in ectatic dilations that in elevated intravascular pressure are incapable of increasing their tone. The varicosities can be uni- or bilateral. In some cases varicosities, first appearing during pregnancy (more often in the second trimester), spontaneously disappear or decrease in the postpartal period.

The patients begin to complain when the disease enters the stage of decompensation: they experience a feeling of heaviness in the legs, and easy fatiguability, sometimes dull pains in the legs, and convulsions of calf muscles (in pregnant women such convulsions can occur due to calcium deficiency caused by increased calcium consumption for the formation of the fetal skeleton). These disorders usually disappear after a night's sleep or after elevation of the legs. In the evening, and especially when the weather is hot, slight (or seldom marked) edema of the ankles and slight swelling of the legs are observed. However, in some cases vein dilations in the lower extremities are accompanied by severe pain limiting a pregnant woman's mobility and sometimes requiring rest and elevation of the legs. In trophic skin disorders the patients complain of itching. Pronounced dilation of vaginal and vulval veins causes a feeling of discomfort; such varicosities practically always completely disappear after labor.

In the compensation stage vein dilation is insignificant or moderate, sometimes segmental. The veins are soft, easily collapsing; the skin over them remains unchanged. In the decompensation stage vein dilation is marked, the veins are tense, and their walls may be sclerotic and fused to the skin. The skin is often pigmented, and trophic disorders develop (initially on the anteromedial surface of the lower legs) that lead to the onset of eczema.

Pregnant women suffering from varicose veins have a high risk of phlebitis, periphlebitis, phlebothrombosis, and thromboembolic complications; ruptures of varicose nodes in the cervix, vagina, and external genitals with the formation of hematomas and bleeding may sometimes be observed (especially during labor). In the puerperium thrombophlebitis is frequent.

Management in pregnancy is nonsurgical: elastic stockings or bandages should be put on before getting up in bed and worn all day long. Discomfort caused by vulvar varicosities can be eliminated or reduced by wearing special support garments. Pregnant women should avoid wearing rolled garters or hose. Oral administration of calcium dobesilate, tribenozide, and similar angioprotectors is recommended; angioprotectors are used locally and leg exercises are performed. Surgical correction (ligation and stripping of varicose veins) is not performed if varicosities first appeared during pregnancy, as venous lesions may disappear some time after labor. In addition, the results of surgical treatment and sclerotherapy are better if they are performed in nonpregnant women. In rare cases surgical interventions may be considered in threatening advance of preexisting varicosities. It should be recognized that in pregnancy, in the condition of increased blood coagulability, the risk of postoperative venous thrombosis is enhanced during vein surgery. Sclerotherapy should be performed with utmost care only by an experienced surgeon in the surgical vascular unit and only when strongly indicated, after a thorough examination of the competency of deep veins of the extremities has been performed. The intervention seems justified only in pronounced functional and trophic (ulcers) disorders and should not be performed after the 34th week of gestation (Wallois 1982). In acute phlebitis of varicose superficial veins, to avoid congestion in the entire leg venous system contributing to the extension of the process to proximal and deep veins, an active walking regimen (Savelyev and Yablokov 1982), elevation of the affected leg in bed and oral administration of antiinflammatory drugs and angioprotectors are recommended. The treatment should be long term. In thrombosis of varicose large saphenous vein, an operation is indicated as a preventive measure against pulmonary artery thromboembolism and the involvement of deep femoral veins into the thrombotic process. In severe varicosities of vulvar and vaginal veins cesarean section may sometimes be necessary.

Pregnancy in uncomplicated varicose vein disease can be retained as a rule if there are no coexisting diseases worsening the maternal prognosis.

14.3 Thrombosis and Thromboembolism in Pregnancy

The mechanism of thromboembolic complications is, to a great extent, related to blood coagulation disturbances; however, vascular wall alterations and peculiarties of blood flow in the altered vessels can play a certain role. Pregnancy affects all three factors. Vascular wall alterations during pregnancy have already been discussed, but as in the majority of cases they do not involve the endothelium their role in the onset of venous thrombosis in pregnant women is doubtful. As to arterial thrombosis, endothelial lesions are accompanied by platelet adhesion to subendothelial collagen, activation of Hageman factor, thrombin formation, platelet aggregation, and, finally, the formation of white thrombus consisting of platelet aggregates and fibrin strips. Pregnancy increases adhesive platelet properties and decreases fibrinolytic blood activity (Handin 1974). Blood congestion in the deep pelvic and leg veins due to the inferior vena cava compression by the uterus can certainly contribute to thrombus formation during pregnancy. Red thrombi forming in the venous system consist of thrombin strips and intermediate erythrocytes. Predisposition to thrombus formation (in the presence of other promoting factors and influences) is enhanced by physiological increase in blood coagulability during pregnancy directed at the prevention of bleeding. Pregnancy and especially labor associated with additional load on hemostatic mechanisms increase the risk of thromboembolic complications in women. In pregnancy, the plasma level of factors VII, VIII, IX, X, and XII rises; fibrinogen and plasminogen content increases; while factor III and XI levels decrease (Chard and Lilford 1983). The changes are directed at increasing fibrin-forming ability (Davis and McNicol 1978). Even in normal pregnancy the plasma contains soluble fibrin monomer complexes, commonly characteristic of prethrombotic or thrombotic conditions. During labor factor VIII plasma level dramatically increases, while the blood clotting time decreases. In the puerperium factor VIII plasma level, fibrinogen content, and platelet count remain increased (Bonnar et al. 1970). The reduction in blood fibrinolytic activity, hypercoagulation, and large tissue thromboplastin stores in the placenta — all form the conditions for the onset of intravascular coagulation.

Thromboembolic complications can pose a serious vital threat in pregnancy and after delivery. Most common in pregnancy are phlebitis, thrombophlebitis, and thrombosis of the deep pelvic veins and the femoral venous system, as well as pulmonary artery embolism; embolisms in other vascular systems (cerebral, mesenteric, carotid) are less frequent. During premature separation of the placenta or embolism by amniotic fluid, disseminated intravascular coagulation may develop.

The incidence of thrombophlebitis during pregnancy compared with the incidence of the disease in nonpregnant women of childbearing age moderately increases; however, in the puerperium the incidence of thrombophlebitis and other thromboembolic complications considerably increases especially after complicated labor or cesarean section and in women receiving estrogen-containing drugs for the suppression of lactation, as well as in obesity and diabetes mellitus. Patients above 40 and those with thromboembolic disease and complications in their history are at higher risk. Pregnancy, on the whole, increases the risk of thromboembolic complications sixfold (Morris and Mitchell 1978). Pregnant women with valvular heart disease, especially when they are accompanied by atrial fibrillation, are at the highest risk (Burch 1977). Atrial fibrillation in women of childbearing age most often accompanies mitral stenosis. According to Villasanta (1965), 19% of pregnant women with untreated deep vein thrombophlebitis develop pulmonary artery embolism, with a 28% lethality.

Pregnant women may rather frequently have phlebothrombosis — noninflammatory pathology caused by blood clot formation partially or completely obstructing the vein lumen. In pregnancy phlebothrombosis can be promoted by venous intima swelling, subintimal accumulation of fibrin, fatty degeneration of the media, slower blood flow in the leg veins, and increased thromboplastin plasma content (Pfeifer 1967). Deep vein thrombosis during pregnancy often reccurs and progresses, and in 50% of cases is complicated by embolisms.

Differential diagnosis of thrombophlebitis and phlebothrombosis is associated with certain difficulties. In thrombophlebitis there is an apparent clinical pattern of acute inflammation; increase of body temperature, chill, malaise, and marked local inflammatory changes. Deep vein thrombosis in the lower extremities in pregnant women is threatened with the onset of the postthrombophlebitic syndrome.

14.3.1 Thrombophlebitis (Venous Thrombosis) of the Inferior Vena Cava System

14.3.1.1 Subcutaneous Vein Thrombophlebitis

Acute thrombophlebitis becomes manifest in pain along the affected vein. The vena saphena magna is most frequently involved while the involvement of the vena saphena parva is less frequent, and the subcutaneous arm veins are least frequently involved (usually as a complication of intravenous drug infusions or blood sampling for laboratory testing). Patients complain of redness, local heat, and tenderness along the course of the subcutaneous vein. On inspection, hyperemia and skin swelling over the inflamed vein can be visible. An indurated and tender vein is palpated, with the sites of thrombus formation thickened. Regional lymphatic nodes are enlarged and painful. Body temperature is either insignificantly increased or normal.

Acute thrombophlebitis of superficial veins can become subacute even without treatment. Subacute thrombophlebitis becomes manifest in slight or moderate spontaneous pains along the occluded vein (which become stronger on palpation) and in vein indurations. In chronic superficial thrombophlebitis pain during walking and vein palpation is insignificant.

14.3.1.2 Deep Vein Thrombophlebitis

Thrombosis of one or two deep crural veins with the patency of other veins maintained causes no serious hemodynamic disturbances and, therefore, can become manifest only in the pains in the calf muscles that become stronger with ankle joint movements (the symptom is relatively pathognomonic if the pain is felt on dorsiflexion of the foot when the leg is bent in the knee); not infrequently palpation of the musculus gastrocnemius is painful. Crural edema may be absent or insignificant (the crural edema and feeling of tension can be present in pregnant women without vein thrombosis). In unilateral phlebitis, asymmetry of the skin temperature can be detected (by electrothermometer). In thrombosis of all deep calf veins there is marked pain, a feeling of inflation, and sometimes foot and crural cyanosis. In femoral vein thrombosis pain and the feeling of muscular tension predominate along the vein. Deep vein thrombophlebitis is commonly accompanied by fever and leukocytosis. A thrombus can be located by the Doppler ultrasound technique.

The clinical pattern of acute ileofemoral vein thrombosis develops within several hours or 1 day. There is an acute pain in the leg, becoming more severe during movement. Body temperature is promptly and significantly elevated. The affected leg becomes swollen, and sometimes there is pudendal lip and buttock edema, the skin surface becoming pale or cyanotic, and tense. Skin palpation (and even mere touching) is very painful; on the first 2–3 days of the edema no dents remain on palpation. The affected vein (posterior tibial, popliteal, femoral) is usually impossible to palpate due to edema and severe pain. In mild thrombosis all these symptoms can be not very marked.

Inadequately treated acute deep thrombophlebitis can assume a subacute form. Leg edema and pain somewhat decrease, body temperature normalizes, and the patient can move her leg and go for short distance walks; however, even insignificant strain enhances the pain and increases the edema.

Chronic deep thrombophlebitis is accompanied by a relatively insignificant leg edema, soft tissues are indurated, and pain on deep palpation along the affected veins and during exercise (walking or prolonged standing) persists; leg edema also increases after exertion, and pain in the muscles of the affected leg is frequently felt.

The feasibility of instrumental diagnosis of venous thrombosis during pregnancy is limited. The ultrasound Doppler technique, impedance, and occlusive plethysmography can be used, while venography and the ^{125}I-labeled fibrinogen test are contraindicated because of the risk of fetal irradiation. The latter procedure should not be performed in the puerperium as well, as free ^{125}I penetrates into the maternal milk. If venography is still to be performed the uterus should be shielded from direct irradiation.

14.3.2 Pulmonary Thromboembolism

Pulmonary thromboembolism is usually a complication of some forms of congenital heart disease, acquired valvular heart disease, and thrombophlebitis; it may arise after surgery on small pelvis organs and in the puerperium. Complete or partial thrombosis regression occurs in 20%–67% of cases.

Depending on the degree and location of obstruction in the pulmonary artery and its branches, clinical manifestations may vary from deteriorated cardiac or pulmonary function in patients with cardiovascular and pulmonary diseases or fever of unclear origin (refractory to therapy with antibiotics) to sudden death.

In massive thromboembolism with circulatory obstruction there is acute anginal chest pain, and shock often develops. Cyanosis, tachypnea, tachycardia, and sometimes distension of the neck veins, hepatic enlargement, and tenderness appear. In pulmonary infarction, tachypnea, tachycardia, fever, cough, hemoptysis, and signs of pleuropneumonia can be observed (muffled percutory sounds, weakened respiration, pleural friction rub, and moist rales), the latter corresponding to zones that are supplied with blood by the obstructed pulmonary artery branches. In circulatory obstruction the murmur peculiar to congenital pulmonary artery stenosis is audible (more often the pulmonic component of the second heart sound may become accentuated), and presystolic gallop is heard. Paroxysms of atrial flutter or fibrillation are rather frequent.

The ECG in pulmonary artery obstruction exhibits a rightward shift of the electrical heart axis, deep S_I wave; transitional zone with rS complex is displaced leftward from V_I to V_4, sometimes V_6; $T_{V_{1-3}}$ wave inversion or right bundle branch block can be noted; deep Q wave and ST segment elevation often occurs in lead III and is less frequent in aVR with concomitant ST segment depression in leads I, aVL and chest leads; and high peaked $P_{II, III}$ waves are often detected. Pulmonary infarction produces no electrocardiographic changes.

Roentgenographic findings indicate sudden interruption of the vascular markings distal to the obstruction of major vessels, greater transparency of the corresponding lung segment or lobe, and increased shadow density of the adjacent segments or the contralateral lung. In pulmonary infarction, the roentgenographic pattern may resemble that of pneumonitis, an area of consolidation with rounded profile appears somewhere on the periphery of the lung, or the roentgenogram may be normal.

The erythrocyte sedimentation rate is commonly increased, and neutrophilic leukocytosis is observed in pulmonary infarction. The blood levels of LDH, SGOT, and fibrin/fibrinogen degradation products are increased.

Pulmonary angiography and lung ventilation-perfusion scintigraphy may, in some cases, appear necessary to confirm the diagnosis.

14.3.3 Leg Artery Thromboembolism

Systemic arterial thromboembolism in pregnancy is usually a complication of mitral sometimes aortic valvular heart diseases, especially the ones accompanied by atrial fibrillation, or less frequently a complication of bacterial endocarditis. Arterial thromboembolism becomes manifest in the onset of acute pain in the extremity and its pallor and coldness, later on cyanotic spots appearing on the skin. Superficial vein collapse is observed. Paresthesia, hypesthesia, and then anesthesia develop. Arterial pulsation is undetectable, muscular weakness gradually developing. If such symptoms are present in both legs, it is indicative of aortic bifurcation embolism; pain in this case can irradiate into the lower abdomen.

14.3.4 Mesenteric Artery Thromboembolism

Mesenteric artery thromboembolism is quite infrequent in pregnancy. Depending on the degree and location of the obstruction, it can be asymptomatic or can be accompanied by dull pain in the abdomen; however, there is sometimes the pattern of acute abdomen. In the latter case, the pain is severe and sudden, and is relieved only by repeated injections of narcotics; it is cramping and can change its localization. Coffee-ground vomiting or diarrhea with blood admixtures are possible. In the first 1–2 h of the disease, the abdomen is soft, and moderately painful on palpation, peristalsis being undetectable. Later on moderate rigidity of the abdominal wall may develop. Collapse can occur.

14.3.5 Cerebral Thromboembolism

Cerebral thromboembolism is a not uncommon complication encountered in pregnancy. It can occur in rheumatic heart disease, bacterial endocarditis, and mitral valve prolapse. In most cases it arises suddenly, after physical exertion or emotional stress, sometimes in acute blood pressure elevation. The appearance of focal neurological disorders without premonitory symptoms in the absence of any or in the presence of signs of mild diffuse cerebral involvement is typical. Neurological disorders depend on the vascular caliber and site of the occlusion. Aphasia, transient localized convulsions, sensitivity disturbances, and monoparesis can appear. Hemiplegia, hemiparesis, and generalized convulsions (of the type of epileptiform fits) can possibly occur.

14.3.6 Treatment of Thrombosis and Thromboembolism

In the acute phase the patients should be kept on bed rest. To relieve pain in acute thrombosis and thromboembolism morphine hydrochloride or pethidine are administered subcutaneously and noramidopyrinmethansulfonate sodium or droperidol is intravenously injected. In the presence of heart or vascular failure the appropriate therapy must be performed.

In acute venous thrombosis anticoagulant therapy with heparin is performed; it seems more expedient (Savelyev and Yablokov 1982) to inject heparin intramuscularly or intravenously (100 U/kg, every 4 h for the first 5–6 days), then the drug dose is reduced every day for 1 week by 1250–2500 U with the same injection frequency. Three to five days before heparin is discontinued coumarin derivatives are given (if not strictly contraindicated). The treatment should be performed under the monitoring of coagulation state by thromboelastography (optimal hypocoagulability is from −4 to −6) and partial thromboplastin time (optimal hypocoagulability from 1 to 2.5 times normal). If anticoagulant therapy is complicated by bleeding, protamine sulfate should be injected if heparin therapy is performed, and fresh blood should be transfused if warfarin therapy is performed (Nesbitt and Abdul-Karim 1982). The use of warfarin is not recommended in pregnancy due to the high risk of fetal hemorrhages, especially during labor. In the latter case it is better to use heparin before labor. Some authors believe it possible to use warfarin in the puerperium (Orme et al. 1977). During the first 7 days low molecular weight dextran (rheomacrodex) at a dose of 1 g/kg daily and a 1% solution of nicotinic acid at a dose of 2–2.5 mg/kg daily should be administered by continuous intravenous drip. It should be recognized that in venous thrombosis streptokinase, streptodekase and urokinase are effective only in the first days (according to the same data, also later) of fresh thrombus formation.

Antibiotics are obligatory if there are signs of infection and especially in suspected septic pelvic thrombophlebitis (Nesbitt and Abdul-Karim 1982).

In pulmonary artery, leg and arm, and cerebral arterial thromboembolism urgent anticoagulant or thrombolytic therapy is required. When thromboembolism is suspected 10000 units heparin should be applied intravenously in a single injection. After the diagnosis is confirmed constant infusions of heparin (1000 units/h) should be continued for 24–28 h or 5000–10000 units of the drug should be administered intravenously every 4 h. The treatment lasts 7–10 days and is regulated by laboratory tests (activated partial thromboplastin time, 60–80 s; clotting time, 20–40 min). Long-term anticoagulant therapy (heparin intramuscularly or subcutaneously or oral anticoagulants) is continued for 6–12 weeks (Bell and Simon 1982; McFadden and Braunwald 1984). In massive thromboembolism, streptokinase may be administered; 250000 units is infused intravenously for 30 min; and then 2000000 to 2500000 units is drip infused for 24 h. During thrombolytic therapy the thrombin time should be two to seven times baseline (Bell and Simon 1982). At completion of streptokinase infusion heparin therapy is to be started. In cerebral arterial thromboembolism the dosage may be approximately half that of the above-mentioned ones.

The treatment with streptokinase, if necessary, may be performed for many days. It should be recognized that streptokinase injections can cause pyrogenic and allergic reactions and profuse uterine bleeding in the early puerperium. Instead of 2500000 to 2750000 U streptokinase, 4400 U/kg per hour of urokinase that is neither pyrogenic nor antigenic can be administered. Though there is an opinion that streptokinase (and especially urokinase) is contraindicated in the early puerperium and in the first 5 months of pregnancy (Hanin et al. 1984), there is also a report on successful use of streptokinase in thrombosis with no side effects either in the mother or fetus (Romani et al. 1982). In pulmonary artery and leg artery thromboembolism, single intravenous injection of 3000000 U streptodekase may prove effective.

Choosing thrombolytic drug doses one should bear in mind that plasma volume in pregnancy is augmented. But in overdosage blood plasma transfusion is preferable to the infusion of aminocapronic acid penetrating through the placenta.

Subcutaneous heparin injections every 8–12 h can be used for the prevention of thromboembolism recurrence. The application of indirect-acting coumarin anticoagulants should be avoided in the first trimester of pregnancy and it should be discontinued 2–3 weeks before labor. After labor heparin or indirect-acting anticoagulant administration should be resumed (Orme et al. 1977). As the risk of thromboembolic complications is especially high in the puerperium, preventive anticoagulant therapy is obligatory in all the women with deep vein thrombosis or pulmonary artery embolism in their history. The treatment with thrombolytic agents and anticoagulants is performed under the monitoring of blood coagulation state.

Pregnant women with acute vein and artery thrombosis of the extremities should be admitted to surgical hospitals (preferably with vascular units). Medical therapy of thromboembolism of small pulmonary artery branches can be performed in high-risk pregnancy units. Embolectomy is possible in pregnant women as well (Gataulin et al. 1979); sometimes it is necessary to perform thrombectomy, plication, or ligation of great veins in surgical (vascular) units. Interruption of the inferior vena cava during pregnancy is also possible (Evans et al. 1968, Savelyev et al. 1979).

Pregnant women with suspected mesenteric artery thromboembolism should be immediately admitted to hospital for urgent surgery. Pregnant women with acute cerebral circulatory disorders should not be transported into neurological or neurosurgical units without special consultations of a neurologist, except for cases when thromboembolism occurred neither at home nor in a medical institution. In cerebral vascular embolism pregnant women should be placed with her head and the upper part of the body elevated. If hospitalization is delayed heparin is administered intravenously by continuous drip first at a dose of 10000–20000 U, with subsequent intramuscular injections of 10000 U every 6 h.

In succesful treatment of thromboembolism termination of pregnancy is not necessary. In recurring thromboembolism the decision is sometimes made to terminate pregnancy. Repeated pregnancies in women who have previously had deep vein thrombosis may be accompanied by the disease recurrence or sometimes by obstetric complications during labor and in the puerperium.

Measures directed at stasis limitation in the leg veins may prevent thromboembolism (and partly vein dilation). Pregnant women should avoid passive standing (walking contributes to venous outflow), lying supine in bed, or sitting with bent knees. To prevent thromboembolism it is also important to eliminate atrial fibrillation, promote early ambulation after labor, and recommend wearing elastic stockings. Women with thromboembolism in their history or those at high risk of thromboembolism are recommended preventive heparin injections for 24 h after delivery (Jackson 1973). Longer preventive therapy of thromboembolism in women with previous thromboembolism in history is sometimes also recommended: anticoagulant therapy is commenced from the 36th week of pregnancy and lasts untill the 6th week of the puerperium (Laros and Alger 1979).

15 Contraception and Sterilization in Cardiovascular Diseases

15.1 Contraception in Cardiovascular Diseases

Contraception (as the basic method of birth control) in some cases helps women with cardiovascular diseases to avoid the risk of death or in other cases aggravation of their condition. In young women with heart and vascular diseases who may be treated surgically or medically contraception helps to avoid undue pregnancy before surgery or effective medical therapy have been performed. It should be recognized that termination of pregnancy is not always safe and sterilization evokes irreversible consequences, sometimes causing psychological trauma. In view of the above, the physician must recommend an adequate method of contraception. Unfortunately, this is not always easy to achieve. Thus, according to Mlczoch et al. (1982) 50% of patients with congenital heart disease do not use any form of contraception, while the majority of those who do resort to contraception take oral contraceptive pills, which is associated with increased risk of complications in many cardiovascular diseases.

The most simple methods of contraception are: interrupted sexual intercourse and periodic abstinence from intercourse on certain days of the menstrual cycle. However, these ways cannot be considered really appropriate, the former making one or both spouses neurotic and the latter (basal body temperature method) being effective only when ovulation is controlled by the regular taking of morning rectal temperature, which most women give up very soon. Calculation of "safe days" by the calender method of Ogino and Knaus is hardly reliable and should not be recommended (Eliseev 1982).

The old barrier method — vaginal insertion of a correctly adjusted occlusive diaphragm, performed carefully by the patient herself with the concomitant use of spermicides (foam, cream, jelly) is relatively effective and absolutely harmless for women with cardiovascular diseases (Taurelle et al. 1976; Arnon and Steinfeld 1985) but still does not give a 100% guarantee of adequate contraception (Kleinman 1983).

Modern mechanical means of contraception are intrauterine devices (coil, loop, bow) inserted by the physician into the uterus for a long period. Correct use of intrauterine devices permits relatively reliable birth control; however, they should be used with caution in women with a number of heart diseases. Pain and considerable blood loss during and sometimes in between menses are not the main contraindications for their use in women with cardiovascular diseases, though abundant blood loss during menses in patients with pulmonary artery stenosis or Eisenmenger's syndrome can give rise to episodes of syncope (Perloff 1984). The presence of a foreign device in the uterus in 20%–75% of cases causes inflammatory changes in the endometrium and cervical tissues, which lead to infection and are responsible for capillary fragility in the upper layers of the endometrium. In view of this, intrauterine contraceptive devices are not to be used in heart and vascular disorders that may be complicated by bacterial infection (bacterial endocarditis in the history, rheumatic mitral and aortic valvular disease, atrial and ventricular septal defects, patent ductus arteriosus, Eisenmenger's syndrome, etc.), as well as in diseases and conditions requiring long-term treatment with anticoagulants (thrombophlebitis, prosthetic cardiac valves, etc.). Intrauterine contraceptive devices seem to be most appropriate in women with arterial hypertension.

Hormonal oral contraceptive pills, the most widespread and willingly used agents, have proved to be not as harmless as expected. Hormonal contraceptives have been shown to reduce tolerance to carbohydrates (which is particularly dangerous for women with diabetes mellitus, as well as for obese women), impair lipid metabolism (additional risk of atherosclerosis development in women with hyperlipoproteinemia), contribute to sodium and water retention, sometimes induce arterial (systemic and pulmonary) hypertension, as a rule increase platelet aggregation ability, decrease fibrinolytic activity, activate the blood coagulation system (which presents a threat of thromboembolism), and attenuate anticoagulation action of coumarin derivatives due to the estrogen effect; with possible neurovegetative dystonia and psychic depression developing (Brenner and Mischell 1975; Taurelle et al. 1976; Kay 1982; Weir 1985; Moser 1986). The incidence of thromboembolic complications (in coronary and cerebral arteries) is higher in women over 25 (and particularly over 40), especially those who smoke (Jaillard 1983). A comprehensive prospective study has shown a higher incidence of pulmonary artery embolism and deep vein thromboembolism in patients taking oral contraceptives (Vessey et al. 1986).

Side effects of hormonal contraceptives are attributed to estrogen action; therefore, estrogen content in modern oral contraceptive drugs is minimal (50 μg and less), or sometimes continuous administration (less effective) of only minimal progestagen doses is used. In the sequential method (not very effective either) estrogen use is followed by the combination of estrogen and progestagen. The combined method (the most effective one — less than 1% of pregnancies) presupposes daily administration of low estrogen and progestagen doses for 3 weeks of the menstrual cycle, the administration beginning from day 5 of the cycle. The investigation conducted in Sweden (Böttiger et al. 1980) has shown that even the reduction of the estrogen content in these preparations fails to decrease mortality due to thromboembolic complications (deep vein thrombosis with pulmonary artery embolism, arterial thromboembolism, including cerebral and coronary). Identical results have been obtained in other investigations (Weir 1985). It is hoped that further perfection of the contraceptive composition will remove their side effects. At present oral contraceptives are contraindicated in arterial hypertension of any etiology, preeclampsia in the history, heart failure (estrogens increase the plasma volume, systolic and cardiac output, and venous return, and impair the water-electrolyte balance), as well as in any diseases threatened with thromboembolic disorders (namely in many forms of congenital cyanotic heart disease, peripartal cardiomyopathy, atrial fibrillation, thrombophlebitis, varicose veins), hyperlipidemia, combinations of cardiovascular diseases with anemia, diabetes mellitus, obesity, and other metabolic disorders. The least number of cardiovascular complications was expected during continuous administration of progestagens, which possess no hypertensive effect (Soutoul and Renaud 1979). However, it should be recognized that progestagens have an anabolic effect, sometimes resulting in undesirable weight gain. In addition, this contraception method often disturbs the menstrual cycle, possibly leading to amenorrhea (Moser 1986). It should also be noted that there was a significant trend toward an increase in cardiovascular morbidity (including ischemic heart disease and stroke) with higher doses of progestagen in combined pills (Meade et al. 1980; Kay 1982). Diuretics sometimes recommended with the use of combined contraceptive help avoid the risk of sodium and water retention but heighten the risk of thrombosis. To reduce the risk of thrombosis anticoagulants should not be used in combination with estrogen-progestagen preparations, as the developing shifts in the blood coagulation system can be hardly monitored and controlled. Drugs containing 50 µg and more of estrogens are absolutely inappropriate in cardiovascular diseases.

Injectable contraceptives (depot-medroxyprogesterone acetate injected once in 3 months) can exert an anabolic effect, raise blood pressure, and disturb the menstrual cycle, which may disorientate the woman and reduce remote efficacy of contraception. In addition, there is a possible risk that depot-medroxyprogesterone acetate may produce persistent infertility (Moser 1986) and possess carcinogenic properties although this is yet to be confirmed.

It should be noted that contraception requires education of women, for incorrect, careless, or irregular use of contraceptives reduces its efficacy.

There are also methods of contraception for males. Correct use of condoms is almost 100% effective. Vasectomy that in recent years has become rather widespread does not seem to be absolutely acceptable for it is practically a sterilizing procedure, though there are reports (Prakash et al. 1980) of successful recanalization of the vas deferens following previously performed vasectomy. Upon recanalization of the vas deferens by microsurgery, fertility is recovered only in 40%–70% of cases (Jarow et al. 1985). The attempts to create contraceptive pills for men affecting spermatogenesis or sperm maturation have so far not yielded any success.

15.2 Sterilization in Cardiovascular Diseases

In certain cases, when even minimal risk of pregnancy is dangerous, sterilization (tube ligation) of a sick woman is advisable. This seems especially expedient if cesarean section is performed on a patient with severe inoperable heart disease, malignant hypertension, or other severe diseases. However, the final decision can be taken by a cardiologist together with a gynecologist only when the patient has given written consent. Surgical sterilization should not be performed right after vaginal delivery or therapeutic abortion, though there are authors who are in favor of sterilization immediately after labor (Rush 1983). A woman with heart disease should be given a rest to be followed by an assessment of the functional state of her cardiovascular system and, if necessary, medical pretreatment before surgical intervention (Nesbitt and Abdul-Karim 1982). It should be recognized that surgical sterilization is associated with a certain risk of thromboembolism in women with cardiovascular diseases threatened with thromboembolic complications. Tube ligation can be performed either using laparotomy or transvaginally (in women with severe heart diseases

Trendelenburg's position in the latter approach should be avoided, this approach being contraindicated in women on continuous anticoagulant therapy). In recent years sterilization has been performed by laparoscopy and electrocoagulation. Experience has shown that bipolar and not unipolar electrocoagulation is preferable (Moser 1986). This method requires an experienced surgeon and the use of pneumoperitoneum, which is not always advisable in severe heart disease (Trendelenburg's position in such cases should also be avoided).

The physician's verdict on the necessity of sterilization is difficult to accept; therefore, it is essential to consider the form and degree of cardiovascular disease, peculiarities of its course and prognosis, possibilities of surgical treatment, the patient's age and number of children in the family, as well as the course of the disease during previous pregnancies and its effect on these pregnancies. In some cases the presence of concomitant (noncardiovascular) diseases can play a decisive role, making pregnancy absolutely contraindicated.

References

Aalkjaer C, Danielsen H, Johannesen P, Pedersen EB, Rasmussen A, Mulvany MJ (1985) Abnormal vascular function and morphology in preeclampsia: A study of isolated resistance vessels. Clin Sci 69: 477–482

Adams JQ (1968) Management of the pregnant cardiac patient. Clin Obstet Gynecol 11: 910–923

Ahronheim JH (1977) Isolated coronary periarteritis. Report of a case of unexpected death in a young pregnant woman. Am J Cardiol 40: 287–290

Allonen H, Kanto J, Iisalo E (1976) The foeto-maternal distribution of digoxin in early human pregnancy. Acta Pharmacol Toxicol (Copenh) 39: 477–480

Altchek S, Albright NL, Somers SC (1968) The renal pathology of toxemia of pregnancy. Obstet Gynecol 31: 595–607

Anichkova ZY (1977) Pregnancy and labour in patients after cardiac surgery. In: Davydov SN (ed) Pregnancy and labour in patients with heart disease (in Russian). Leningrad Institute for Advanced Medical Training, Leningrad, pp 35–42

Aoi W, Doi Y, Tasaki S, Mitsuoka T, Suzuki S, Hashiba K (1978) Primary aldosteronism aggravated during peripartum period. Jpn Heart J 19: 946–953

Arias F, Pineda J (1978) Aortic stenosis and pregnancy. J Reprod Med 20: 229–232

Arnon RG, Steinfeld L (1985) Medical management of the cyanotic patient with congenital heart disease. Cardiovasc Rev Rep 6: 146–156

Asmussen I (1978) Arterial changes in infants of smoking mothers. Postgrad Med J 54: 200–204

Asmussen I (1979) Fetal cardiovascular system as influenced by maternal smoking. Clin Cardiol 2: 246–252

Assali NS, Brinkman CR (1972) Disorders of maternal circulatory and respiratory adjustments. In: Assali NS (ed) Pathophysiology of gestation, vol I. Maternal disorders. Academic, New York, pp 269–353

Auinger W (1967) Schwangerschaft bei erworbenen und angeborenen Herzklappenfehlern. Wien Z Inn Med 48: 353–360

Avar Z, Toth B, Matos J, Zacher P (1976) Früh- und Späteffecte des Gestationverlaufes nach Kommisurotomien. Zentralbl Gynakol 98: 833–847

Bader ME, Bader RA (1968) Cardiovascular hemodynamics in pregnancy and labor. Clin Obstet Gynecol 11: 924–939

Baskin CG, Law S, Wenger NK (1980) Sulfadiazine rheumatic fever prophylaxis during pregnancy: does it increase the risk of kernicterus in newborn? Cardiology 65: 222–225

Batson GA (1974) Cyanotic congenital heart disease and pregnancy. Br J Obstet Gynaecol 81: 549–553

Bauer TW, Moore GW, Hutchins GM (1982) Morphologic evidence for coronary artery spasm in eclampsia. Circulation 65: 255–259

Bay W, Ferris TF (1979) Factors controlling plasma renin and aldosterone during pregnancy. Hypertension 1: 410–415

Becker RM (1983) Intracardiac surgery in pregnant women. Ann Thorac Surg 36: 453–458

Bekker SM (1975) The pathology of pregnancy (in Russian). Meditsina, Leningrad

Belch JMF, Thorburn J, Greer IA, Safro S, Prentice CRM (1985) Intravenous prostacyclin in the management of pregnancies complicated by severe hypertension. Clin Exp Hypertens (B) 4: 75–86

Bell WR, Simon TL (1982) Current status of pulmonary thromboembolic disease. Pathophysiology, diagnosis, prevention, and treatment. Am Heart J 103: 239–262

Bellet S (1972) Essentials of cardiac arrhythmias. Diagnosis and management. Sanders, Philadelphia

Berglund F, Fledh H, Lunborg P, Prame B, Sannerstedt R (1984) Drug use during pregnancy and

breast-feeding. A classification system for drug information. Acta Obstet Gynecol Scand (Suppl) 126: 1–55
Bergman AS (1976) The role of etilefrine in the complex therapy of arterial hypotension in pregnancy (in Russian). Vopr Okhr Mater Det 9: 55–59
Bergman AS (1983) Vascular dystonia and pregnancy (in Russian). Zinatne, Riga
Berke RA, Hoops EC, Kereiakes JC, Saenger EL (1973) Radiation dose to breast-feeding child after mother has ^{99m}Tc-MAA lung scan. J Nucl Med 14: 51–52
Biale Y, Cantor A, Leventhal H, Gueren M (1980) The course of pregnancy in patients with artificial heart valves treated with dipyridamole. Int J Gynaecol Obstet 18: 128–132
Bieniarz J, Crottogini JJ, Curuchet E, Romero-Salinos G, Yoshida T, Poseiro JJ, Caldeyro-Barcia R (1968) Aortocaval compression by the uterus in late human pregnancy. II. An arteriographic study. Am J Obstet Gynecol 100: 203–217
Biggs JSG (1975) Blood pressure changes following smoking in pregnancy. Aust NZ J Med 15: 204–208
Biglieri EG, Slaton PE (1967) Pregnancy and primary aldosteronism. J Clin Endocrinol 27: 1628–1632
Bloshansky YM (1974) Fetal and newborn health care in extragenital diseases of the mother (in Russian). In: Proceedings of the X National Congress of Pediatrics, Moscow, pp 12–13
Bonnar J, McNicol GP, Douglas AS (1970) Coagulation and fibrinolytic mechanisms during and after normal childbirth. Br Med J 2: 200–203
Borima TA, Pakhmurny BA, Vaniyev PA (1977) Changes in watersalt metabolism and their role in the pathogenesis of heart failure in pregnant women (in Russian). Akush Ginecol (Mosk) 3: 22–25
Bornstein A, Dalal P, Tischler J, Novack S, Michaelson S (1984) Acute myocardial infarction in a thirty-six year old postpartum female. Angiology 35: 591–594
Böttiger LE, Boman G, Eklund G, Westerholm B (1980) Oral contraceptives and thromboembolic disease. Effects of lowering oestrogen content. Lancet 1: 1097–1101
Braunwald E (1984) Valvular Heart Disease. In: Braunwald E (ed) Heart Disease. A Textbook of Cardiovascular Medicine. Saunders, Philadelphia, pp 1063–1135
Brenner PF, Mishell DR Jr (1975) Contraception for the woman with significant cardiac disease. Clin Obstet Gynecol 18: 155–168
Brock R (1952) Valvotomy in pregnancy. Proc R Soc Med 45: 538–540
Broughton-Pipkin F, Symonds EM, Turner SR (1982) The effect of captopril (SQ 14,255) upon mother and fetus in the chronically cannulated ewe and pregnant rabbit. J Physiol 323: 415–422
Brown AK, Doukas N, Riding WD, Jones EW (1967) Cardiomyopathy and pregnancy. Br Heart J 29: 387–393
Burakovsky VI, Vanina LV, Bokeria LA, Beylin AL, Pankratova NN, Kostyukov VV (1976) Hyperbaric oxygenation in the management of labour in patients with severe congenital heart disease (in Russian). Akush Ginecol 8: 8–10
Burch GE (1977) Heart disease and pregnancy. Am Heart J 93: 104–116
Burg JR, Dodek A, Kloster FE, Metcalfe J (1974) Alterations of systolic time intervals during pregnancy. Circulation 49: 560–564
Buxbaum A, Aygen MM, Shahin W, Levy MJ, Ekerling B (1971) Pregnancy in patients with prosthetic heart valves. Chest 50: 639–642
Campbell M (1965) Causes of malformations of the heart. Br Med J 2: 895–904
Carruth JE, Mirvis SB, Bregan DR, Wenger NK (1981) The electrocardiogram in normal pregnancy. Am Heart J 106: 1075–1078
Casanegra P, Aviles G, Maturana G, Dubernet J (1975) Cardiovascular management of pregnant women with a heart valve prosthesis. Am J Cardiol 36: 802–806
Casarotto D, Bortolotti U, Russo R, Betti D, Schivazappa L, Thiene G (1979) Surgical removal of left atrial myxoma during pregnancy. Chest 75: 390–392
Cavanagh D, Rao PS, Tuny K, Gaston LW (1972) Toxemia of pregnancy. The development of an experimental model in the primate. Obstet Gynecol 39: 637–638
Caves PK, Paneth M (1972) Acute mitral regurgitation in pregnancy due to ruptured chordae tendinae. Br Heart J 34: 541–544
Chard T, Lilford R (1983) Basic sciences for obstetrics and gynaecology. Springer, Berlin Heidelberg New York

Chebotarev DF (1960) Internal diseases in obstetric and gynecological practice (in Russian). Zdorovye, Kiev

Chervenak FA, Berkowitz RL (1985) Hypertension in pregnancy. Mt Sinai J Med 52: 46–58

Chesebro JH, Fuster V, Elveback LR, McGoon DC, Pluth JR, Puga FJ, Wallace R, Danielson GK, Orszulak TA, Pichler JM, Schaff HV (1983) Trial of combined warfarin plus dipyridamole or aspirin therapy in prosthetic heart valve replacement: danger of aspirin compared with dipyridamole. Am J Cardiol 51: 1537–1541

Chesley LC (1978) Hypertensive disorders in pregnancy. Appleton-Century-Crofts, New York

Chesley LC (1980) Severe rheumatic cardiac disease and pregnancy: the ultimate prognosis. Am J Obstet Gynecol 136: 552–558

Chesley LC, Duffus GM (1971) Posture and apparent plasma volume in late pregnancy. J Obstet Gynaecol Br Commonw 78: 406–412

Chesley LC, Talledo E, Bohler CS, Zuspan FD (1965) Vascular reactivity to angiotensin II and norepinephrine in pregnant and nonpregnant women. Am J Obstet Gynecol 91: 837–842

Chesley LC, Annito JE, Cosgrove RA (1976) The remote prognosis of eclamptic women. Sixth periodic report. Am J Obstet Gynecol 124: 446–459

Cibils LA (1974) The placenta and newborn infant in hypertensive conditions. Am J Obstet Gynecol 118: 256–270

Clark SL, Phelan JP, Creenspoon J, Aldhal D, Horenstein Y (1985) Labor and delivery in the presence of mitral stenosis. Central hemodynamic observations. Am J Obstet Gynecol 152: 984–988

Cohen WR, Steiman T, Patsner B, Snyder D, Satwicz P, Monroy P (1983) Acute myocardial infarction in a pregnant woman at term. JAMA 16: 2179–2181

Collins JH, Gomes G, Brown JW, Muller R (1985) Infective endocarditis presenting with a pneumothorax in a patient 32 weeks pregnant. J La State Med Soc 157: 60–63

Collins R, Yusuf S, Peto R (1985) Overview of randomized trials of diurectics in pregnancy. Br Med J 290: 17–23

Comino-Delgado R (1984) Influence of the body position on taking blood pressure. Clin Exp Hypertens (B) 3: 75–83

Conradsson TB, Werkö L (1974) Management of heart disease in pregnancy. Progr Cardiovasc Dis 16: 407–420

Cooley DA, Chapman DW (1952) Mitral commissurotomy during pregnancy. JAMA 150: 113–1114

Cottrill CM, McAlister RG, Gettes L, Noonan JA (197)) Propranolol therapy during pregnancy, labor and delivery. J Pediatr 91: 812–817

Crane MG, Andes JP, Harris JJ, Slate WG (1964) Primary aldosteronism in pregnancy. Obstet Gynecol 23: 200–208

Cšapo A (1950) Actomyosin formation by estrogen action. Am J Physiol 162: 406–410

Cutforth R, MacDonald CB (1966) Heart sounds and murmurs in pregnancy. Am Heart J 71: 741–747

Danforth DN (1982) Other complications and disorders due to pregnancy. In: Danforth DN (ed) Obstetrics and Gynecology, 4th edn. Harper and Row Philadelphia, pp 475–494

Dattino M, Niccoli V, Dattino R (1986) Metodi di diagnostica delle cardiopatie in gravidanza. Clin Ter 116: 237–241

Davies JA, McNicol JP (1978) Blood coagulation and thrombosis. Br Med Bull 34: 113–121

Davis JE, Leider HJ (1977) Rupture of prosthetic graft of aorta in pregnancy. Am J Obstet Gynecol 124: 397–399

Davydov SN, Anichkova ZY, Varavko EZ, Samorodinova LA (1977) The effect of pregnancy and labour on the natural history of heart disease. In: Davydov SN (ed) Pregnancy and labour in patients with heart disease (in Russian). Leningrad Institute for Advanced Medical Training, Leningrad, pp 5–10

Deeg P (1983) Herzerkrankungen bei Frauen in gebärfähigen Alter. Dtsch Arztbl 80: 48–52

Demakis JG, Rahimtoola SH, Sutton GC, Meadows WR, Szanto PB, Tobin JR, Gunnar LM (1971) Natural course of peripartum cardiomyopathy. Circulation 44: 1053–1061

Dementyeva MP, Lyakhov NG, Timoshek ZN, Majdan GP (1975) A case of myocardial infarction in a pregnant woman (in Russian). Klin Med (Mosk) 10: 141–143

Demidov VN (1976) Syndrome of the inferior vena cava compression (in Russian). Vopr Okhr Mater Det 10: 78–81

Demidov VN, Fuks MA (1976) A case of echocardiographic pericardial cyst diagnosis in pregnancy (in Russian). Kardiologiia 9: 138–139

Denbow CE, Matadial L, Sivapragasam S, Spencer H (1983) Pregnancy in patients after homograft cardiac valve replacement. Chest 83: 540–542
Dequiedt P, Cotteel M, Legras-Turquet V, Turquet M, Beneit O, Leblen J, Dracon M, Puech F (1984) Données epidemiologique sur l'hypertension arterielle gravidique. J Gynecol Obstet Biol Reprod (Paris) 13: 889–896
De Swiet M (1976) Pregnancy and maternal heart disease. Br J Hosp Med 15: 353–360
Diamond MA, Murray RH, Schmid P (1970) Idiopathic postural hypotension. Physiologic observations and report of a new mode of therapy. J Clin Invest 49: 1341–1348
Didia TG, Dzhvebenava GG, Bakradze MM, Katamadze TV, Batiashvili DD (1983) Efficiency of laser treatment in pregnant patients with arterial hypotension (in Russian). Akush Ginekol (Mosk) 12: 15–17
Dubois D, Petitcolas J (1978) Beta-bloquants et grossesse á hauts risques. Point de vue du néphrologue et de l'obstetricien. Nouv Presse Med 7: 2811–2812
Dubois D, Petitcolas J, Temperville B, Kiepper A, Catherine P (1983) Beta blocker therapy in 125 cases of hypertension during pregnancy. Clin Exp Hypertens (B) 2: 41–59
Duminy PC, Burger PD (1981) Fetal abnormality associated with the use of captopril during pregnancy. S Afr Med J 60: 805–805
Eliahou HE, Silverberg DS, Reisin E, Romem I, Mashiach S, Serr DM (1978) Propranolol for the treatment of hypertension in pregnancy. Br J Obstet Gynaecol 85: 431–436
Eliseev OM (1975) Heart disease and pregnancy (in Russian). Kardiologiia 2: 143–153
Eliseev OM (1979) Arterial hypertension in pregnancy (in Russian). Ter Arkh 8: 134–139
Eliseev OM (Jelissejev OM) (1981) Arterielle Hypertonie bei Schwangeren. In: Fruhman B, Heberer G, Jelissejev O, Rudolf W, Zander J (eds) Aktuelle Probleme der Gesundheitsfursorge. Urban and Schwarzenberg, Munich, pp 340–343
Eliseev OM (1982) Cardiovascular system and pregnancy. In: Chazov El (ed) Handbook of Cardiology (in Russian). Meditsina, Moscow, vol 4, pp 350–394
Engel HJ, Engel E, Lichtlen PR (1983) Coronary atherosclerosis and myocardial infarction in young women — role of oral contraceptives. Eur Heart J 4: 1–8
Esscher EB (1981) Congenital complete heart block in adolescence and adult life. A follow-up study. Eur Heart J 2: 281–288
Etheridge MJ (1969) Heart disease and pregnancy. Aust NZ J Obstet Gynaecol 9: 7–10
Evans G, Dallen JE, Dexter L (1968) Pulmonary embolism during pregnancy. JAMA 206: 320–326
Evans-Jones JC (1983) Hypertrophic cardiomyopathy in pregnancy. J R Soc Med 76: 524–525
Finnerty FA (1977) Hypertension in pregnancy. Angiology 28: 535–544
Finnerty FA (1980) Hypertension and pregnancy. J Cardiovasc Med 5: 559–569
Foidart JM, Rorive G (1977) Hypertension of grossesse. Acta Cardiol (Brux) 32: 187–202
Friedberg CK (1963) Diseases of the heart, 3rd edn. Sanders, Philadelphia
Fujita K, Yamasaki S, Tamaki N (1978) Cerebro-vascular accident during pregnancy. No Shinkei Geka 6: 989–995
Gallery EDM (1980) Modern management of hypertension in pregnancy. Aust NZ J Med 10: 246–252
Gallery EDM, Ross M, Hunyor SN, Györy AZ (1977) Predicting the development of pregnancy-associated hypertension. The place standardized blood pressure measurements. Lancet I: 1273 to 1275
Garden A, Davey DA, Dommisse Y (1982) Intravenous labetolol and intravenous dihydralazine in severe hypertension in pregnancy. Clin Exp Hypertens (B) I: 371–383
Gataulin NG, Mukhometrakhimov FF, Yarullina FY, Semenov II (1979) Embolectomy in pulmonary artery thromboembolism (in Russian). Grudn Khir 2: 76–78
Gembitsky EV (1982) Neurocirculatory hypotension and hypotensive conditions. In: Chazov EI (ed) Handbook of cardiology (in Russian). Meditsina, Moscow, pp 101–117
Gerbert G (1986) Herzinfarkt vermehrt bei Frauen. Orale Kontrazentive erhöhen bei Raucherinnen das Risiko kardiovaskularer Komplikationen. Fortschr Med 104: 20–21
Ginz B (1970) Myocardial infarction in pregnancy. J Obstet Gynecol 77: 610–615
Gladstone GR, Hordof A, Gersony WM (1975) Propranolol administration during pregnancy. Effects on the fetus. J Pediatr 86: 962–968
Glebova VV, Estifaev NN, Kaluzhina VS, Vlasova AB (1972) Acute pulmonary edema in pregnant women with heart disease. In: Rodionov VV, Serov VN (eds) Clinical pattern, diagnosis and

management of emergencies (in Russian). Moscow Medical Stomatological Institute, Moscow, pp 68–70
Gleicher N, Meller J, Sandler RZ, Sallum S (1981) Wolff-Parkinson-White syndrome in pregnancy. Obstet Gynecol 58: 748–752
Goeschen K, Schmoldt V, Pluta M, Saling E (1985) Einfluß eines niedrigen Blutdruckes auf die Venenfunktion in und außerhalb der Schwangerschaft und therapeutische Konsequenzen. Geburtshilfe Frauenheilkd 45: 525–533
Gogin EE, Senenko AN, Tyurin EI (1983) Arterial hypertensions (in Russian). Meditsina, Leningrad
Goodwin JF (1961) Pregnancy and coarctation of the aorta. Clin Obstet Gynecol 4: 645–664
Goodwin JF (1982) The frontiers of cardiomyopathies. Br Heart J 48: 1–18
Gordon RD, Fishman LM, Liddle JW (1967) Plasma renin activity and aldosterone secretion in a pregnant woman with primary aldosteronism. J Clin Endocrinol 27: 385–388
Gore I, Seiwert VJ (1952) Dissecting aneurysm of the aorta. Pathologic aspects: Analysis of 85 fatal cases. Arch Pathol 53: 121–141
Gormley MJJ, Hadden DR, Murnaghan GA, Sheridan B, Montgomery DAD (1982) Cushing's syndrome in pregnancy. Clin Endocrinol 16: 283–293
Grand A, Barrillon A (1976) Infarctus myocardique et grossesse. Coeur Med Interne 15: 345–358
Grimes EM, Fayez JA, Miller GL (1973) Cushing's syndrome and pregnancy. Obstet Gynecol 42: 550–559
Grünberger W, Leodolter S, Parschalk O (1978) Schwangerschaftshypotension der Einfluss von Mineralkortikoiden auf die fetale Ernährung. Geburtsh Frauenheilkd 38: 1070–1074
Haas JM (1976) The effects of pregnancy on the midsystolic click and murmur of the prolapsing posterior leaflet of the mitral valve. Am Heart J 92: 407–408
Hadden DR (1982) Endocrine and metabolic disorders. Clin Obstet Gynecol 9: 29–57
Haites NE, McLennan FM, Movat DHR, Rawles JM (1985) Assessment of cardiac output by the Doppler ultrasound technique alone. Br Heart J 53: 123–129
Hall JG, Pauli RM, Wilson KM (1980) Maternal and fetal sequelae of anticoagulation during pregnancy. Am J Med 68: 122–140
Hamilton BE (1947) Report from the cardiac clinic of the Boston lying-in hospital for the first twenty-five years. Am Heart J 33: 663–668
Hamilton HFH (1950) Symposium of hemodynamics in pregnancy, cardiac output in pregnancy. Edinburgh Med J, March, 1–9
Handin RJ (1974) Thromboembolic complications of pregnancy and oral contraceptives. Progr Cardiovasc Dis 16: 395–400
Hanin B, Julien J, Gaillard JL, Samama M (1984) Controversies about thrombolytic therapy. Int Angiol 3: 343–353
Hankins GDV, Wendel GD, jr, Leveno KG, Stoneham J (1985) Myocardial infarction during pregnancy: review. Obstet Gynecol 65: 139–146
Hartz SC, Heinonen OP, Shapiro S, Siskind V, Slone D (1975) Antenatal exposure to meprobamate and chlordiazepoxide in relation to malformation, mental development, and childhood mortality. N Engl J Med 292: 726–728
Hausen WJ, Loch EG (1973) Bedeutung von Herzkrankheiten während der Schwangerschaft. Z Allgemeinmed 49: 995–998
Hawkins DF (1976) Teratogens in the human. Current problems. J Clin Pathol, suppl 10: 150–156
Hayslett JP, Lynn RI (1980) Effects of pregnancy in patients with lupus nephropathy. Kidney Int 18: 207–220
Hendriks CH, Quilligan EJ (1956) Cardiac output during labor. Am J Obstet Gynecol 71: 953–972
Hirsh J, Cade JF, O'Sullivan EF (1970) Clinical experience with anticoagulant therapy during pregnancy. Br Med J I: 270–273
Hirsch J, Cade JF, Gallus (1972) Anticoagulants in pregnancy. A review of indications and complications. Am Heart J 83: 301–305
Hou SH, Grossman SD, Medias NE (1985) Pregnancy in women with renal disease and moderate renal insufficiency. Am J Med 78: 185–194
Howie PW, Begg CB, Purdie DW, Prentice CRM (1976) Use of coagulation test to predict the clinical progress of preeclampsia. Lancet II: 323–325
Howitt G (1971) Heart disease and pregnancy. Practitioner 206: 765–772

Hunyor SH (1984) Vascular volume and cardiac response to normal and hypertensive pregnancy. Hypertension 6, suppl III: III-128–III-132
Hytten FE, Leitch I (1964) The physiology of human pregnancy. Davis, Philadelphia
Hytten FE, Thomson AM (1968) Water and electrolytes in pregnancy. Br Med Bull 24: 15–18
Iams JD, Rayborn WF (1982) Drug effects on the fetus. In: Rayborn WF, Zuspan FP (ed) Drug therapy in obstetrics and gynecology. Appleton-Century-Crofts, Norwalk, pp 9–17
Ibarra-Perez C, Arevalo-Toledo N, Alvarez-de la Cadena OA, Noriega-Guerra L (1976) The course of pregnancy in patients with artificial heart valves. Am J Med 61: 504–512
Ingemarsson I, Liedholm H, Montan S, Westren M, Melander A (1984) Fetal heart rate during treatment of maternal hypertension with beta-adrenergic antagonists. Acta Obstet Gynecol Scand suppl 118: 95–97
Ingram RH, Braunwald E (1984) Pulmonary edema: cardiogenic and noncardiogenic. In: Braunwald E (ed) Heart disease. A textbook of cardiovascular medicine, vol 1. Saunders, Philadelphia, pp 560–577
Ishikawa K, Matsuura S (1982) Occlusive thromboaortopathy (Takayasu's disease) and pregnancy. Clinical course and management of 33 pregnancies and deliveries. Am J Cardiol 50: 1293–1300
Jackson P (1973) Puerperal thromboembolic disease in "high risk" cases. Br Med J I: 263–264
Jacoby WJ Jr (1964) Pregnancy with tetralogy and pentalogy of Fallot. Am J Cardiol 14: 866–873
Jaillard J (1983) Les accidents artériels de la contraception per oestro-progestatifs. Ann Med Interne (Paris) 134: 416–420
Jaluvka V (1970) Herzkrankheiten und Müttersterblichkeit. Gynaekol Rundsch 10: 209–240
Jankowski CB (1986) Radiation and pregnancy. Putting the risks in proportion. Am J Nurs 86: 260–265
Jarow JP, Budin RE, Dym M, Zirkin BR, Noren S, Marshall FF (1985) Quantitative pathologic changes in the human testis after vasectomy. A controlled study. N Engl J Med 313: 1252–1256
Jonáš V (1960) Clinical cardiology (in Russian). State Medical Publishers, Prague
Jones AM, Howitt G (1965) Eisenmenger syndrome in pregnancy Br Med J I: 1627–1631
Jorde A, Morack G (1970) Herzkrankheiten in Verbindung mit Schwangerschaft und Geburt. Zentralbl Gynaekol 92: 169–175
Julian DJ, Szekely P (1985) Peripartum cardiomyopathy. Progr. Cardiovasc Dis 27: 223–240
Kahhale S, Carrara W, Barros ACSD, Zungaib M, Neme B (1984) A comparative study between treated (beta-blocker pindolol) and untreated hypertension. Clin Exp Hypertens (B) 3: 171
Kaluzna J (1977) Evaluation of the effect of pregnancy on the efficiency of the cardiovascular system in women with acquired valvular heart disease (in Polish). Kardiol Pol 20: 207–212
Karim SMM, Hillier K, Somers K, Trussell RR (1971) The effects of prostaglandins E_2 and $F_{2\alpha}$ administered by different routes on uterine activity and the cardiovascular system in pregnant and non-pregnant women. J Obstet Gynaecol Br Commonw 78: 172–179
Katz R, Karliner JS, Resnik R (1978) Effects of a natural volume overload state (pregnancy) on left ventricular performance in normal human subjects. Circulation 58: 434–441
Kay CR (1982) Progestagens and arterial disease — evidence from the Royal College of General Practitioner's Study. Am J Obstet Gynecol 142: 762–765
Kereni TD, Gleicher N, Meller J, Brown E, Steinfeld L, Chitkara U, Raucher H (1980) Transplacental cardioversion of intrauterine supraventricular tachycardia with digitalis. Lancet II: 393–394
Kincaid-Smith P (1975) The kidney clinico-pathological study. Blackwell Scientific, Oxford
Kincaid-Smith P, Fairley KF (1976) The differential diagnosis between preeclamptic toxemia and glomerulonephritis in patients with proteinuria during pregnancy. In: Lindheimer MD, Katz AI, Zuspan FP (eds) Hypertension in pregnancy. Wiley, New York, pp. 157–166
Kirushchenkov AP (1978) The effect of harmful factors on the fetus (in Russian). Meditsina, Moscow
Kleinman RL (1983) Periodic abstinence for family planning. IPPF Medical, London
Kochar MS, Itzkovitz HD (1978) Treatment of idiopathic orthostatic hypotension (Shy-Drager syndrome) with indomethacin. Lancet I: 1011–1014
Kofler E, Gerstner G, Huber J(1982) Antikonzeption, Schwangerschaft und Entbindungsmethoden bei angeborenen und erworbenen Vitien. Herz/Kreisl 6: 355–359
Kolibash AJ, Ruiz DE, Lewis RP (1975) Idiopathic hypertrophic subaortic stenosis in pregnancy. Ann Intern Med 82: 791–798
Korenevskaya IL (1978) Hemodynamics in pregnant patients with mitral stenosis (in Russian). Kardiologiia 2: 122–126

Korolev BA, Karov VV, Gomozova IA (1986) Surgical treatment of pregnant patients with rheumatic mitral stenosis (in Russian). Revmatologiia (Moskva) 1: 3–5

Kovatz S, Arber I, Korzets Z, Pathaus M, Ben Aderet N, Bernheim J (1985) Urinary kallikrein in normal pregnancy, pregnancy with hypertension and toxemia. Nephron 40: 48–51

Kozdoba OA (1970) Diagnosis of various forms of pregnancy-associated hypertension (in Russian). Kardiologiia 7: 98–104

Krausz Y, Naparstek E, Eliakim M (1978) Idiopathic pericarditis and pregnancy. Aust NZ J Obstet Gynaecol 18: 86–89

Krayenbühl HP, Siegenthaler W (1974) Schwangerschaft bei Herzkranken. Med Klin 69: 321–324

Kremkau EL, Gilbertson PR, Bristow JD (1973) Acquired, nonrheumatic mitral regurgitation: clinical management with emphasis on evaluation of myocardial performance. Progr Cardiovasc Dis 15: 403–425

Kuchel O, Buu NI, Gutkowska J, Genest J (1980) Treatment of severe orthostatic hypotension by metoclopramide. Ann Intern Med 93: 841–843

Kulago GV (1974) On the characteristics of the incidence of hypotensive conditions (in Russian). Zdrav Belorusii 4: 38–42

Kunz J, Schreiner WE (1982) Pharmakotherapie während Schwangerschaft und Stillperiode. Thieme, Stuttgart

Kunz J, Zogg M (1980) Beitrag zur Betreuung von Schwangeren mit Herzvitien. Schweiz Med Wochenschr 110: 674–684

Kusche M, Bolte A, Hollmann W, Roemer D (1986) Körperliche Leistungsfähigkeit im Verlauf der Schwangerschaft. Geburtsh Frauenheilk 46: 151–156

Kuzmenko ZP (1980) Ways of enhancing adaptive abilities in the pregnant patients with rheumatic valvular heart disease (in Russian). Akush Ginekol (Mosk) 6: 36–38

Laros RK, Alger LS (1979) Thromboembolism and pregnancy. Clin Obstet Gynaecol 22: 871–887

Lauckner W, Schwarz R, Retzke U (1978) Die Eignung von Mephentermin zur Behandlung der arteriellen Hypotonie in der Schwangerschaft. Zentralbl Gynaekol 100: 217–221

Laurens P, Gavelle P, Farge C, Dubost Cl, Maurice Ch (1983) Stimulation cardiaque isotopique et maternités. Apropos de 25 observations. Arch Mal Couer 76: 733–738

Lauritzen C (1985) Medikamente während der Gravidität. Diagnostik 18: 16–21

Lauritzen C (1986) Arzneimittel während Schwangerschaft und Laktation. Zentralbl Gynaekol 108: 137–154

Lebedeva LI, Orlov LS (1965) On the mechanisms of atrioventricular block in healthy women during labour (in Russian). Kazan Med Zh 2: 22–25

Legostayev AF, Drozdov MI (1978) The effect of complex therapy on the course of pregnancy and labour in patients with arterial hypotension (in Russian). In: Abstracts of a symposium on Pregnancy and extragenital pathology, Orel, pp 48–49

Lepp Y, Karma K (1978) On the course of some adaptive cardovascular reactions in pregnancy (in Russian). In: Riyo J (ed) Modern problems of Cardiology. Tartu University Press, Tartu, pp 87–89

Lequime J, Doumit J, Rolis O (1970) The role of environment in the aetiology of congenital heart disease. Z Kreislaufforsch 59: 559–565

Levis P (1983) Peripartuale Kardiomyopathie. Schweiz Med Wochenschr. 113: 373–375

Lewis RB, Schulman JD (1973) Influence of acetylsalicylic acid on inhibitor of prostaglandin synthesis, on the duration of human gestation and labour. Lancet II: 1159–1161

Leyse R, Ofstun M, Dillard DH, Merendino K (1961) Congenital aortic stenosis in pregnancy corrected by extracorporeal circulation, offering a viable male infant in term, but with anomalies eventuating in his death at four months of age. JAMA 176: 1009–1012

Lieber S, Dewilde P, Huyghens L, Traey E, Gepts E (1985) Eisenmenger's syndrome and pregnancy. Acta Cardiol (Brux) 40: 421–424

Lieberman BA, Stirrat GM, Cohen SL, Beard RW, Pinker GD (1978) The possible adverse effect of propranolol on the fetus in pregnancies complicated by severe hypertension. Br J Obstet Gynaecol 85: 678–683

Lighter ES, Allen HD, Loughlin G (1977) Neonatal hyperthyroidism and heart failure. A differential approach. Am J Dis Child 131: 68–70

Limacher MC, Ware JA, O'Meara ME, Fernandez GC, Young JB (1985) Tricuspid regurgitation

during pregnancy: two-dimensional and pulsed Doppler echocardiographic observations. Am J Cardiol 55: 1059–1062
Lin CC, Lindheimer MD, River P, Moawad AH (1982) Fetal outcome in hypertensive disorders of pregnancy. Am J Obstet Gynecol 142: 255–260
Lind J, van Papendrecht H (1984) Obstetrical complications in a patient with the Marfan syndrome. Eur J Obstet Gynecol Reprod Biol 18: 161–168
Lindberg BoS, Sandström Bo (1981) How Swedish obstetricians manage hypertension in pregnancy. A questiannaire study. Acta Obstet Gynecol Scand 60: 327–331
Lindmark G, Lindberg B, Högstedt S (1984) The incidence of hypertensive disease in pregnancy. Acta Obstet Gynecol Scand suppl 118: 29–32
Little B (1965) Water and electrolyte balance during pregnancy. Anesthesiology 26: 400–408
Lo Cicero G, Cellina G, Binaghi P, Limonta A (1985) Validita della metodica ecocardiografica nella determinazione della gettata sistolica in corso di gravidanza. Minerva Cardioangiol 33: 187–190
Lubbe WF (1984) Hypertension in pregnancy. Pathophysiology and management. Drugs 28: 170–188
Lunnell NO, Nylund L, Lewander R, Sarby B, Wager J (1984) Uteroplacental blood flow in pregnancy hypertension after the administration of a beta-adrenoceptor blocker, pindolol. Gynecol Obstet Invest 18: 269–274
Lutz DJ, Noller KL, Spittell JA, jr (1978) Pregnancy and its complications following cardiac valve prostheses. Am J Obstet Gynecol 131: 460–468
Maarek-Charbit M, Corone P (1986) Syndrome d'Eisemenger et grossesse. Arch Med Coeur 79: 733–740
McAnulty JH, Metcalfe J, Ueland K (1982) Heart disease and pregnancy. In: Hurst W (ed) The heart, 5th edn. McGraw-Hill, New York, pp 1521–1540
McCans JL, Wenger NK (1976) Problems in management of the pregnant patient with rheumatic heart disease and valve prosthesis. South Med J 69: 1007–1010
McCausland AM, Hyman C, Winsor T, Trotter AD (1961) Venous distensibility during pregnancy. Am J Obstet Gynecol 81: 472–479
McComb JM, McNamee PT, Sinnamon DG, Adgey AA (1982) Staphylococcal endocarditis presenting as meningitis in pregnancy. Int J Cardiol 1: 325–327
McFadden ER, Braunwald E (1984) Cor pulmonale and pulmonary thromboembolism. In: Braunwald E (ed) Heart disease. Saunders, Philadelphia
McGrady GA, Daliny JR, Peterson DR (1985) Maternal urinary tract infection and adverse fetal outcomes. Am J Epidemiol 121: 377–381
McKenna WJ, Harris I, Rowland E, Whitelaw A, Storey G, Holt D (1983) Amiodarone therapy during pregnancy. Am J Cardiol 51: 1231–1233
McMahon B, Alpert M, Salber EJ (1966) Infant weight and parental smoking habits. Am J Epidemiol 82: 247–261
MacNab G, Macafee CAJ (1985) A changing pattern of heart disease associated with pregnancy. J Obstet Gynecol 5: 139–142
Majdan JF, Walinsky P, Cowchock SF (1983) Coronary artery bypass surgery during pregnancy. Am J Cardiol 52: 1145–1146
Makolkin VI (1977) Acquired valvular heart disease (in Russian). Meditsina, Moscow
Malbranche-Aupecle MH, Mavel A, Jahier J, Vamp A, Feldman JP (1985) Grossesse chez une patiente porteuse d'un pacemaker atomique pour bloc auriculo-ventriculaire chirurgical apres cure d'une tetralogie de Fallot. A propos d'un cas. Revue de la litterature. Rev Fr Gynecol Obstet 80: 105–107
Mann JI, Inman WHW, Thorogood M (1976) Oral contraceptive use in older women and fatal myocardial infarction. Br Med J II: 445–447
Marsoni V (1985) Effective treatment of post-partum hypotension with dimetophrine. A placebo-controlled, double-blind trial. Curr Med Res Opin 9: 578–585
Mashkovsky MD (1984) Drugs. Meditsina, Moscow
Massobrio M, Benedetto C, Bertini E, Tetta C, Camussi G (1985) Immune complexes in preeclampsia and normal pregnancy. Am J Obstet Gynecol 152: 578–583
Mattoras R, Reque JA, Usandizaga JA, Minguez JA, Larrea JL, Nuñez L (1985) Prosthetic heart valve and pregnancy. A study of 59 cases. Gynecol Obstet Invest 19: 21–31
Mazhdrakov G, Popov N (1976) Diseases of the kidney (in Bulgarian). Meditsina i Phizcultura, Sofia

Meade TW, Greenberg G, Thompson SG (1980) Progestagens and cardiovascular reactions associated with oral contraceptives and a comparison of the safety of 50- and 30 μg oestrogen preparations. Br Med J I: 1157–1161
Meadows WR (1960) Post-partum heart disease. Am J Cardiol 6: 788–802
Melvin KR, Richardson PJ, Olsen EGL, Daly K, Jackson G (1982) Peripartum cardiomyopathy due to myocarditis. N Engl J Med 307: 731–734
Mendelson CL (1960) Cardiac disease in pregnancy. Davis, Philadelphia
Mengert WF, Tacehi DA (1961) Pregnancy toxemia and sodium chloride. Am J Obstet Gynecol 81: 601–605
Metcalfe J, Ueland K (1974) Maternal cardiovascular adjustments to pregnancy. Progr Cardiovasc Dis 16: 363–374
Metcalfe J, Ueland K (1978) The heart and pregnancy. In: Hurst JW (ed) The heart, 4th edn. McGraw-Hill, New York, pp 1721–1755
Meyer MB, Tanascia JA (1977) Maternal smoking, pregnancy complications and perinatal mortality. Am J Obstet Gynecol 128: 494–502
Miniely R, Yuzpe AA, Drake CG (1979) Subarachnoid hemorrhage secondary to ruptured cerebral aneurysm in pregnancy. Obstet Gynecol 53: 64–70
Mlczoch J, Mayr H, Schlemmer M, Mannheimer E (1982) Zur Frage von Schwangerschaften bei Patientinnen mit kongenitalen Herzfehlern. Herz/Kreisl. 6: 350–354
Mochizuki M, Maruo T, Motoyama S (1986) Treatment of hypertension in pregnancy by a combined drug regimen including captopril. Clin Exp Hypertens (B) 5: 69–78
Mok CK, Boey J, Wang R, Chan TK, Cheung KL, Lee PK, Chew J, Ng RP, Tse TF (1985) Warfarin versus dipyridamole-aspirin and pentoxifylline-aspirin for the prevention of prosthetic heart valve thromboembolism: a prospective randomized clinical trial. Circulation 72: 1059–1063
Morris GK, Mitchell JRA (1978) Clinical management of venous thrombo-embolism. Br Med Bull 34: 169–175
Moser W (1986) Moderne Aspekte der Kontrazeption. Wien Med Wochenschr 136: 286–298
Motté G, Vogel M, Coatantiec G, Mariette P, Welti JJ (1975) Thrombose coronarienne aiguë chez une femme de 28 ans. Arch Mal Coeur 68: 91–96
Murdoch JL, Walker BA, Halpern BI, Kuzma JW, McKusick VA (1972) Life expectancy and causes of death in the Marfan syndrome. N Engl J Med 286: 804–808
Murnaghan GA (1982) Cardiovascular disorders and hypertension. Clin Obstet Gynaecol 9: 59–74
National Research Council, Committee on the Biological Effect of Ionizing Radiation (1980) The effects on populations of exposure to low levels of ionizing radiation. National Academy Press, Washington DC, pp 477–514
Neilson G, Galea EG, Blunt A (1970) Congenital heart disease and pregnancy. Med J Aust 1: 1086 to 1088
Nelson MM, Forfar JO (1971) Associations between drugs administered during pregnancy and congenital abnormalities of the fetus. Br Med J 1: 523–528
Nesbitt REL, Abdul-Karim RW (1982) Coincidental disorders complicating pregnancy. In: Danforth WJ (ed) Obstetrics and gynecology, 4th edn. Harper and Row, Philadelphia, p 495–554
Newman RA, Gallager JC, Clements JP, Krakoff IH (1978) Demonstration of Ga-67 localization in human placenta. J Nucl Med 19: 504–506
Nora JJ, Dodd PF, McNamara DG, Hattwick MAW, Leachman RD, Cooley DA (1969) Risk of offspring of parents with congenital heart defects. JAMA 209: 2052–2053
Novy MJ, Edwards MJ (1967) Respiratory problems in pregnancy. Am J Obstet Gynecol 99: 1024 to 1045
Novy MJ, Peterson EN, Metcalfe J (1968) Respiratory characteristics of maternal and fetal blood in cyanotic congenital heart disease. Am J Obstet Gynecol 100: 821–828
Oakley C, Doherty P (1976) Pregnancy in patients after valve replacement. Br Heart J 38: 1140–1148
Oakley GDG, McGarry K, Limb DG, Oakley CM (1979) Management of pregnancy in patients with hypertrophic cardiomyopathy. Br Med J I: 1749–1750
Onrot J, Goldberg MR, Hollister AS, Biaggioni I, Robertson RM, Robertson D (1986) Management of chronic orthostatic hypotension. Am J Med 80: 454–464
Orme ML, Levis PJ, de Swiet M, Serlin MJ, Sibeon R, Baty JD, Breckenridge AM (1977) May mothers given warfarin breastfeed their infants? Br Med J 18: 1564–1565

Palushchinskaya NA, Zhemkauskayte IA, Stoshkute EP (1981) Pregnancy and labour in women with prosthetic cardiac valves (in Russian). Kardiologiia 1: 91–93

Pankratova NN (1974) Anesthesia during cesarean section in patients with heart disease (in Russian). Thesis, First Medical Institute, Moscow

Papi L, Ciustarini C, Filice M, Ballestra AM (1985) Crisi ipertensiva in corso di gestosi E.P.H. trattata con nifedipina per via sublingvale. Minerva Cardioangiol 33: 639–642

Pavlova SS (1974) Comparative assessment of various techniques of general anesthesia during forceps delivery in patients with heart disease (in Russian). Vopr Okhr Mater Det 5: 67–71

Penn IM, Barrett PA, Pannikote V, Barnaby PF, Campbell JB, Lyons NR (1985) Amiodarone in pregnancy. Am J Cardiol 56: 196–197

Pepperell RJ (1983) Drugs in pregnancy. Med Int 1: 1636–1638

Perloff JK (1984) Pregnancy and cardiovascular disease. In: Braunwald E (ed) Heart disease, 2nd edn. Sanders, Philadelphia, pp 1763–1781

Persianinov LS, Bodyazhina VI, Gurtovoy BL (eds) (1978) Handbook of obstetrics and gynecology (in Russian). Meditsina, Moscow

Persianinov LS, Demidov VN (1977) Circulatory function during pregnancy, labour and puerperium. Meditsina, Moscow

Persianinov LS, Chernukha EA, Guriev TD (1978) Late termination of pregnancy with prostaglandin $F_{2\alpha}$ and its analogue 15-methyl PGE_2. In: Markov KM (ed) Prostaglandins in the experiment and clinical practice (in Russian). USSR Ministry of Public Health, Moscow, pp 105–107

Petrovsky BV, Vanina LV, Efuni SN, Beylin AL, Giorgobiani TN, Kretova NE (1981) Hyperbaric oxygenation in the management of labour in patients with congenital and acquired heart disease (in Russian). Vestn Akad Med Nauk USSR 10: 67–72

Pettifor JM, Benson R (1975) Congenital malformations associated with the administration of oral anticoagulants during pregnancy. J Pediatr 86: 459–462

Pfeifer GW (1967) Thromboembolische Komplikationen bei Schwangeren und die thrombolytische Therapie. Therapiewoche 17: 2021–2029

Pirani B, MacGillivray I (1975) The effect of plasma retransfusion on the blood pressure in the puerperium. Am J Obstet Gynecol 121: 221–226

Pitcher D, Leather MH, Storey GCA, Holt DW (1983) Amiodarone in pregnancy. Lancet I: 597–598

Pitts JA, Crosby WM, Basta IL (1977) Eisenmenger's syndrome in pregnancy. Does heparin prophylaxis improve the maternal mortality rate? Am Heart J 93: 321–326

Plotti G, Tropeano G, Colucci P, Gianolla F, Zecchi P, Moneta E (1985) Il prolass della mitrale e la gravidanza. Minerva Med 76: 2007–2010

Pokálev GM (ed) (1974) Neurocirculatory dystonia (in Russian). Volgo-Vyatskoye, Gorky

Pontonnier G, Grandjean H, Sarramon MF, Degoy J, Guiraud R, Favretto R (1975) Chronic fetal distress: research on placental blood flow and therapy. In: Salvadori B (ed) Therapy of fetoplacental insufficiency during pregnancy. Springer, Berlin Heidelberg New York, vol 1, pp 251 to 256

Prakash OM, Grewal PS, Sworgari HK (1980) Recanalization of vas. A study of 25 cases. Antiseptic 77: 397–400

Probst RE, Mier TM (1963) Acute pericarditis complicating pregnancy. Report of a case. Obstet Gynecol 22: 393–395

Protopopova TA (1981) Genetic indexes in women with congenital heart disease and their offsprings (in Russian). Akush Ginekol (Mosk) 10: 17–19

Quilligan EJ (1982) Maternal Physiology. In: Danforth DN (ed) Obstetrics and gynecology. Harper and Row, Philadelphia, pp 326–341

Rakut VS (1981) Hypotension in pregnancy and its effect on the fetus and newborn. In: Fruhmann G, Heberer G, Jelisejew O, Rudolph W, Zander J (eds) Aktuelle Probleme der Gesundheitsfürsorge in Arbeitsmedizin, Kardiologie, Chirurgie, Gynäkologie und Geburtshilfe. Urban and Schwarzenberg, Munich, pp 381–383

Ratner NA (1974) Arterial hypertension (in Russian). Meditsina, Moscow

Rayburn WF, Fontana ME (1981) Mitral valve prolapse and pregnancy. Am J Obstet Gynecol 141: 9–11

Reichek, N, Shelburne JC, Perloff JK (1973) Clinical aspects of rheumatic valvular disease. Progr Cardiovasc Dis 15: 491–537

Retzke U, Schwarz R (1976) Does pregnancy change the regulatory mechanisms in low-pressure system (in Russian). Akush Ginekol (Mosk) 1: 52–55
Rimbach E, Heiligenstein E (1967) Die klinische Bedeutung der Hypotonie in der Schwangerschaft und während der Geburt. Med Welt 18: 1950–1954
Roberts WC (1970) The congenitally bicuspid aortic valve. A study of 85 autopsy cases. Am J Cardiol 26: 72–83
Roberts WC (1981) Aortic dissection. Anatomy, consequences and causes. Am Heart J 101: 195–214
Robson DJ, Jeeva Raj MV, Storey GCA, Holt DW (1985) Use of amiodarone during pregnancy. Postgrad Med J 61: 75–77
Romani A, Chiche G, Elios A, Serradimigni A (1982) Thrombose veineuse de la grossesse. Arteres Veines 1: 371–375
Rosenberg L, Miller DR, Kaufman DW, Helmrich SP, Van de Corr S, Stolley PD, Shapiro S (1983) Myocardial infarction in women under 50 years of age. JAMA 250: 2801–2806
Rotmensch HH, Elkayam U, Frishman W (1983) Antiarrhythmic drug therapy during pregnancy. Ann Intern Med 98: 487–497
Rovinsky JJ, Jaffin H (1965) Cardiovascular hemodynamics in pregnancy. I. Blood and plasma volumes in multiple pregnancy. Am J Obstet Gynecol 93: 1–15
Rovinsky JJ, Jaffin H (1966a) Cardiovascular hemodynamics in pregnancy. II. Cardiac output and left ventricular work in multiple pregnancy. Am J Obstet Gynecol 95: 781–786
Rovinsky JJ, Jaffin H (1966b) Cardiovascular hemodynamics in pregnancy. III. Cardiac rate, stroke volume, total peripheral resistance, and central blood volume in multiple pregnancy. Synthesis of results. Am J Obstet Gynecol 95: 787–794
Rubin SA, Brundage B, Mayer W, Chatterjee K (1979) Usefulness of Valsalva maneuver and cold pressor test for evaluation of arrhythmias in long QT syndrome. Br Heart J 42: 490–492
Rubin PC, Butters L, Clark DM, Reynolds B, Sumner DJ, Steedman D, Low RA, Reid JL (1983) Placebo-controlled trial of atenolol in treatment of pregnancy-associated hypertension. Lancet I: 431–434
Rubin PC, Butters L, Clark D, Sumner D, Belfield A, Pledyer D, Low RAJ, Reid JL (1984) Obstetric aspects of the use in pregnancy-associated hypertension of the β-adrenoceptor antagonist atenolol. Am J Obstet Gynecol 150: 389–392
Rubler S, Hammer N, Schneebaum R (1973) Systolic time intervals in pregnancy and the postpartum period. Am Heart J 86: 182–188
Rubler Sh, Prabodhkumar MD, Pinto ER (1977) Cardiac size and performance during pregnancy estimated with echocardiography. Am J Cardiol 40: 534–540
Rugh R (1969) X-ray overdose cause for abortion. In: Symposium on radiation biology of the fetal and juvenile mammal, Richland, Washington
Rush RW (1983) Cardiac disease in pregnancy. Med Int 1: 1634–1635
Rybkina NF (1960) Heart disease and pregnancy (in Russian). Gorky Book Publishers, Gorky
Samborskaya EP, Gutman LB (eds) (1984) Essential concepts of nutrition in pregnancy (in Russian). Zdorovye, Kiev
Samorodinova LO (1971) Pregnancy and labour in patients with cyanotic valvular heart disease. In: Davydov SN (ed) Pregnancy and labour in patients with heart disease (in Russian). Leningrad Institute for Advanced Medical Training, Leningrad, pp. 27–31
Samorodinova LA, Khantemirova RA, Groshchenkova LB (1971) Pregnancy and labour in patients with congenital acyanotic heart disease. In: Davydov SN (ed) Pregnancy and labour in patients with heart disease (in Russian). Leningrad Institute for Advanced Medical Training, Leningrad pp 21–26
Samoylova GS, Smirnova AA, Voskresenskaya IS (1979) The response of heart work in patients with heart disease on the administration of prostaglandin $F_{2\alpha}$ during induction of abortion in the second trimester of pregnancy (in Russian). In: Abstracts, 3rd congress of obstetrics and gynecology of the Belorussian SSR, Minsk, pp 213–215
Sanderson J, Koech D, Iha D, Ojiambo HP (1985) T-lymphocytes subsets in idiopathic dilated cardiomyopathy. Am J Cardiol 55: 755–758
Sasse L (1975) Transmural myocardial infarction during pregnancy. Am J Cardiol 35: 448–452
Saveleyev VS, Yablokov EG (1982) Diseases of the veins. In: Chazov EI (ed) Heart and vascular diseases (in Russian). Meditsina, Moscow, pp 270–305 (Handbook of cardiology, vol 4)

Saveleyev VS, Yablokov EG, Kiriyenko AP (1979) Pulmonary artery thromboembolism (in Russian). Meditsina, Moscow
Schaedel H, Albert M, Huth JH, Knorre GH, Leutritz, Plass R, Püschel KS, Roboff W (1977) Schwangerschaft und Geburt unter Therapie mit elektrischen Herzschrittmachern. Dtsch Gesundheitswesen 32: 2197–2200
Schaefer G, Arditi LI, Solomon HA (1968) Congenital heart disease and pregnancy. Clin Obstet Gynecol 11: 1048–1063
Schatz IJ (1980) Current management concepts in orthostatic hypotension. Arch Intern Med 140: 1152–1154
Schenker JG, Chowers I (1971) Pheochromocytoma and pregnancy. Review of 89 cases. Obstet Gynecol Surv 26: 739–747
Schroeder, JC, Harrison DC (1971) Repeated cardioversion during pregnancy: treatment of refractory paroxysmal atrial tachycardia during 3 successive pregnancies. Am J Cardiol 27: 445–446
Schwartz DB, Schamroth L (1979) The effect of pregnancy on the frontal plane QRS axis. J Electrocardiography 12: 279–281
Schwarz R (1964) Das Verhalten des Kreislaufs in der normalen Schwangerschaft. II Mitteilung. Arch Gynecol 199: 663–670
Shaffer AB (1975) Congenital heart disease. In: Silber EN, Katz LN (eds) Heart disease. Macmillan, New York, pp 565–696
Shaffer AB, Silber EN (1975) Rheumatic fever and rheumatic heart disease. In: Silber EN, Katz LN (eds) Heart disease. Macmillan, New York, pp 697–758
Serment H, Ruf H (1968) Les dangers pour le produit de conception de médicaments administrés a la femme enceinte. Bull Féd Soc Gynecol Obstet 20: 69–98
Serov VN, Dayanov FV, Smirnova LI (1978) The role of extragenital pathology in terminal conditions during pregnancy and labour. In: Serov VN (ed) Pregnancy and extragenital pathology (in Russian). Regional Medical Office, Orel, pp 7–9
Shah DM, Sunderji SG (1985) Hypertrophic cardiomyopathy and pregnancy. Report of a maternal mortality and review of literature. Obstet Gynecol Surv 40: 444–448
Shapiro EP, Trimble EL, Robinson JC, Estruch MT, Gottlieb SH (1985) Safety of labor and delivery in women with mitral valve prolapse. Am J Cardiol 5: 806–807
Shaver PJ, Carrig TF, Baker WP (1978) Postpartum coronary artery dissection. Br Heart J 40: 83–86
Shekhtman MM (1980) Renal disease and pregnancy (in Russian). Meditsina, Moscow
Shekhtman MM, Barkhatova TP (1982) Internal diseases and pregnancy (in Russian). Meditsina, Moscow
Shekhtman MM, Glezer GA (1978) Hemodynamics and renal function in pregnant patients with hypertension (in Russian). Kardiologiia 11: 77–84
Shrestna NK, Arora R, Padmavati S (1979) Multiple pregnancies in a patient with Fallot's tetralogy. Indian Heart J 31: 58–60
Silber EN, Katz LN (1975) Heart disease. Macmillan, New York
Skryabina EN (1984) On phasic left ventricular hypodynamia syndrome in pregnancy (in Russian). Vrach Delo 5: 73–77
Smirnova LM (1975) Pregnancy and the Adams-Stokes syndrome. In: Sergievsky VP (ed) Modern problems of cardiology, part 2 (in Russian). Kasakhstan Alma-Ata, pp 92–93
Smith DW (1966) Dysmorphology (teratology). J Pediatr 69: 1150–1169
Smith FW, Adam AH, Phillips WDP (1983) NMR imaging in pregnancy. Lancet 1: 61–62
Smith SL, Douglas BH, Langford HG (1967) A model of preeclampsia. II. Changes in renin content produced by anti-placenta serum. Johns Hopkins Med J 120: 220–224
Sokolow M, McIllroy MB (1981) Clinical cardiology, 3rd edn. Lange Medical, Los Altos, pp 714–723
Soradi I (1970) On the content of drugs in breast milk (in Russian). Hungarian Pharmacol 1: 3–8
Soutoul JH, Renaud M (1979) Problèmes posès par la régulation des naissances chez les cardiaques et les hypertendues. Ann Cardiol Angiol 28: 419–422
Spargo BH, Lichtig C, Luger AM, Katz AI, Lindheimer MD (1976) The renal lesion in preeclampsia. In: Lindheimer MD, Katz AI, Zuspan FP (eds) Hypertension in pregnancy. Wiley, New York, pp 129–137
Spargo B, McCartney CP, Winemiller R (1959) Glomerular capillary endotheliosis in toxemia of pregnancy. Arch Pathol 68: 593–599

Speroff L (1973) Toxemia of pregnancy. Mechanism and therapeutic management. Am J Cardiol 32: 582–591

Stanaszek WF, Kellermann D, Brogden RN, Romankiewicz JA (1983) Prazosin update. A review of its pharmacological properties and therapeutic use in hypertension and congestive heart failure. Drugs 25: 339–384

Stevenson RE, Burton M, Ferlauto G, Taylor HA (1980) Hazards of oral anticoagulants during pregnancy. JAMA 243: 1549–1551

Stenstrom G, Swolin K (1985) Pheochromocytoma in pregnancy. Experience of treatment with pheoxybenzamine in three patients. Acta Obstet Gynecol Scand 64: 357–361

Stirrat GM (1976) Prescribing problems in the second half of pregnancy and during lactation. Obstet Gynecol Surv 31: 1–7

Stjerfeldt M, Berglund K, Lindsten J, Ludvigsson J (1986) Maternal smoking during pregnancy and rise of childhood cancer. Lancet I: 1350–1352

Suc JM, Gassia JP, Orfila C, Durand D (1978) L'hypertension arterielle gravidique. Conceptions actuelles. Arch Mal Coeur 71: 30–38

Sugrue D, Blake S, Troy P, MacDonald D (1980) Antibiotic prophylaxis against infective endocarditis after normal delivery — is it necessary? Br Heart J 44: 499–502

Sukerman-Voldman E (1982) Pindolol therapy in pregnant hypertensive patients. Br J Clin Pharmacol 13, suppl. 2: 379–379

Sullivan JM (1974) Blood pressure elevation in pregnancy. Progr Cardiovasc Dis 16: 375–394

Sullivan JM, Ramanathan KB (1985) Management of medical problems in pregnancy — severe cardiac disease. N Engl J Med 313: 304–309

Szekely P, Snaith L (1974) Heart disease and pregnancy. Churchill Livingstone, Edinburgh

Szekely P, Turner R, Snaith L (1973) Pregnancy and the changing pattern of rheumatic heart disease. Br Heart J 35: 1293–1303

Takeda S, Kida H, Yoschimura M, Yokoyama H, Koshino Y, Asamoto T, Tomosugi H, Abe T, Hattori N (1985) Organic glomerular lesions in toxemia of pregnancy. Jpn J Nephrol 27: 803–813

Tanz RD (1963) Inotropic effects of certain steroids upon heart muscle. Rev Can Biol 22: 147–157

Taurelle R, Duhon R (1976) Cardiopaties et grossesse. Deuxiéme partie. La gestation chez les cardiaques. Coeur Med Interne 15: 27–35

Taurelle R, Simon P, Ruet C (1976) Cardiopathies et grossesses. Troisiéme partie. La planification des naissances chez les cardiaques. Coeur Med Interne 15: 189–197

Ticconi C, Valli E, Manna C, Piccione E (1985) Possibilita e limiti dell'impiego dei farmaci betabloccanti nella terapia dell'ipertensione arteriosa in gravidanza. Clin Ter 115: 497–501

Titchenko LI (1985) Mitral valve prolapse syndrome and pregnancy (in Russian). Sov Med 9: 69–74

Titchenko LI (1986) Left ventricular function in pregnant women with aortic valve disease (in Russian). Akush Ginekol (Mosk) 3: 63–66

Tomono S, Ohshima S, Hatori M, Yamamoto S, Li T, Murata K (1982) Vectorcardiographic studies on pregnant women with special referrence to the effect on postural changes. Kitakanto Med J 32: 377–384

Travyanko TD, Khominskaya ZB, Dashkevich VE (1981) Hormonal status in women with rheumatic heart disease in late pregnancy (in Russian). Akush Ginekol (Mosk) 10: 14–16

Tuchmann-Duplessis H (1975) Drug effects on the fetus. Adis, New York

Tuimala RJ, Hertikainen-Sorri AL (1984) Treatment of hypertension during pregnancy by beta blocking agents. Clin Exp Hypertens (B) 3: 167–167

Tulenov MT (1976) Cardiological tactics in pregnant patients with heart disease (in Russian). Kazakhstan, Alma-Ata

Turner AF (1975) The chest radiography in pregnancy. Clin Obstet Gynecol 18: 65–74

Ueland K, Hansen JM (1969) Maternal cardiovascular dynamics II. Posture and uterine contractions. Am J Obstet Gynecol 103: 1–7

Ueland K, Gills RE, Hansen J (1968) Maternal cardiovascular dynamics. I. Cesarean section under subarachnoid block anesthesia, Am J Obstet Gynecol 100: 42–54

Ueland K, Novy MJ, Peterson EN, Metcalfe J (1969) Maternal cardiovascular dynamics. IV. The influence of gestational age on the maternal cardiovascular response to posture and exercise. Am J Obstet Gynecol 104: 856–864

Ueland K, Hansen J, Eng M, Kalappa R, Parer JT (1970) Maternal cardiovascular dynamics. V.

Cesarean section under thiopental nitrous oxide and succinylcholine anesthesia. Am J Obstet Gynecol 108: 615–622
Ueland K, Akamatsy TJ, Eng M, Bonica JJ, Hansen JM (1972) Maternal cardiovascular dynamics. VI. Cesarean section under epidural anesthesia without epinephrine. Am J Obstet Gynecol 114: 775–780
Ueland K, Novy MJ, Metcalfe J (1979) Cardiorespiratory response to pregnancy and exercise in normal women and in patients with heart disease. Am J Obstet Gynecol 115: 4–10
Upshaw CB (1970) A study of maternal electrocardiograms recorded during labor and delivery. Am J Obstet Gynecol 107: 17–27
Vanina LV (1971) Pregnancy and labour in acquired valvular and congenital heart disease (in Russian). Meditsina, Moscow
Vanina LV (1977a) The management of patients with rheumatic heart disease (in Russian). Kardiologiia 1: 147–151
Vanina LV (1977b) Pregnancy and heart disease (in Russian). Akush Ginekol (Mosk) 3: 64–69
Vanina LV (1979) Prospects for reducing the risk of pregnancy and labour in patients with valvular heart disease (in Russian). Vopr Okhr Mater Det 5: 52–58
Vanina LV, Smirnova LM (1978) Pregnancy in patients with prosthetic cardiac valves (review) (in Russian). Med Refer J, Sect 10, 7: 1–8
Vanina LV, Chumak TF, Guseva NA (1976) A technique of rheumatic fever activity determination in the gestational and postpartal periods by cytological examination of milk and colostrum (in Russian). Probl Revmatol 3: 69–71
Vanina LV, Pavlova SS, Pankratova NN (1977) Anesthesiologic management during labour in patients with valvular heart disease (in Russian). Akush Ginekol (Mosk) 1: 30–33
Vanina LV, Kosach GA, Smirnova LM, Rozenfeld LI (1979) Pregnancy in patients with prosthetic cardiac valves (in Russian). Akush Ginekol (Mosk) 11: 23–26
Vanina LV, Glezer IM, Guseva NA (1980) Determination of rheumatic fever activity by immunofluorescent examination of breast milk (in Russian). Akush Ginekol (Mosk) 2: 15–18
Vasilenko VK (1972) Acquired valvular heart disease (in Russian). Zdorovye, Kiev
Vessey M, Mant D, Smith A, Yeates D (1986) Oral contraceptives and venous thromboembolism: findings in a large prospective study. Br Med J 292: 526–526
Villasanta U (1965) Thromboembolic disease in pregnancy. Am J Obstet Gynecol 93: 142–160
Vitushkina GV, Popova AE (1977) Pregnancy and labour in patients with aortic heart disease. In: Davydov SN (ed) Pregnancy and labour in patients with heart disease (in Russian). Leningrad Institute for Advanced Medical Training, Leningrad, pp 16–21
Vogler H (1968) Hypotone Regulationstörungen in Wochenbett und deren Behandlung. Med Welt 19: 2661–2666
Voronin KV, Shekhtman MM, Smirnov VA (1986) Differential approach to diagnosis and treatment of pregnancy-associated arterial hypotension (in Russian). Akush Ginekol (Mosk) 6: 52–54
Wallace WA, Harken DE, Ellis LB (1971) Pregnancy following closed mitral valvuloplasty: a long-term study with remarks concerning the necessity for careful cardiac management JAMA 217: 297–304
Wallenburg HCS, Dekker GA, Makowitz JW, Rotmans P (1986) Low-dose aspirin prevents pregnancy-induced hypertension and pre-eclampsia in angiotensin-sensitive primigravidae. Lancet I: 1–3
Wallois P (1982) Les abus du traitment sclerosant. Phlébologie 35: 789–798
Walsh JJ, Burch GE, Black WC, Fetnans VJ, Hibbs RG (1965) Idiopathic myocardiopathy of the puerperium (postpartal heart disease). Circulation 32: 19–31
Walsh SW (1985) Preeclampsia: An imbalance in placental prostacyclin and thromboxane production. Am J Obstet Gynecol 152: 335–340
Walters BNJ, Redman CWG (1982) Control of severe hypertension in pregnancy with nifedipine. In: Proceedings of the 3rd congress of the International Society of Hypertension in Pregnancy, Dallas, Texas, p 196
Wang RYC, Tam V, Tse T (1982) Pregnancy in Takayasu's arteritis. In: Abstracts of IX world congress of cardiology, vol I, No 0858
Wang RYC, Pui Kee Lee, Chow JSF, Chen WC (1983) Efficacy of low-dose, subcutaneously administered heparin in treatment of pregnant women with artificial heart valves. Med J Aust 2: 126 to 128

Weiner CP, Sokol ML, Vaisrub N (1984) Control of preeclamptic hypertension by ketanserin — a serotonin receptor antagonist. Am J Obstet Gynecol 149: 496–500

Weir RJ, Brown JJ, Fraser R, Kraszewski A, Lever AF, McIlwaine GM, Morton JJ, Robertson JIS (1973) Plasma renin, renin substrate, angiotensin II and aldosterone in hypertensive disease of pregnancy. Lancet I: 291–294

Weir RJ (1985) Blood pressure and the contraceptive pill. In: Bulpitt CJ (ed) Epidemiology of hypertension. Elsevier Science, Amsterdam, pp 289–300 (Handbook of hypertension, vol. 6)

Wellen I (1953) Infant mortality in specific hypertensive disease of pregnancy and in essential hypertension. Am J Obstet Gynecol 66: 36–45

Wenderlein JM (1976) „Kreislaufbeschwerden" in der Schwangerschaft. Herz/Kreisl 8: 625–628

Wenger NK (1978) Myocardial involvement in systemic disease. In: Hurst W (ed) The heart. McGraw-Hill, New York, pp 1590–1635

Wenner L (1979) Varikosis, Hormone, Schwangerschaft. Vasa 8: 258–262

White WB (1984) Management of hypertension during lactation. Hypertension 6: 297–300

Whittemore R, Hobbins JC, Engle MA (1982) Pregnancy and its outcome in women with and without surgical treatment of congenital heart disease. Am J Cardiol 50: 641–651

Wicker P, Dallocchio M (1984) Alpha-bloquants en hypertension arterielle. Bordeaux Med 17: 974–978

Wohlert M, Solling J, Pedersen EB, Johannesen P, Kristensen S, Lauritsen JG, Rasmussen AB (1984) Circulating immune complexes and hypertension in pregnancy. Acta Obstet Gynecol Scand 63: 609–611

World Health Organization (1984) Cardiomyopathies, Technical Report Series 697

Zakirov IZ, Shakirov DZ, Mardanov LM (1979) Pregnancy and rheumatic fever (in Russian). Meditsina, Tashkent

Zatikyan EP (1983) Changes in venous return in pregnancy (in Russian). Krovoobrasheniie 3: 44–47

Zelenin VF (1962) Heart disease and pregnancy. In: Lukomsky PE, Savitsky NN (eds) Handbook of internal diseases (in Russian). Meditsina, Moscow, vol I, pp 482–486

Zierler S, Rotman KJ (1985) Congenital heart disease in relation to maternal use of bendectin and other drugs in early pregnancy. N Engl J Med 313: 347–352

Zimmerman J, Shotan A (1984) Prosthetic valve endocarditis in pregnancy. Acta Obstet Gynecol Scand 63: 731–732

Zipes DP (1984) Specific arrhythmias: Diagnosis and treatment. In: Braunwald E (ed) Heart disease. A textbook of cardiovascular medicine. Saunders, Philadelphia, pp 683–743

Zitnik RS, Branderburg RO, Sheldon MD, Wallace RB (1969) Pregnancy and open-heart surgery. Circulation 39, suppl. I: 257–262

Zucker MD, Peterson J (1970) Effect of acetylsalicylic acid, other non-steroidal antiinflammatory agents and dipyridamole on human blood platelets. J Lab Clin Med 76: 66–75

Zuspan FP (1984) Chronic hypertension in pregnancy. Clin Obstet Gynecol 27: 854–873

Subject Index

FSC
www.fsc.org
MIX
Papier aus verantwortungsvollen Quellen
Paper from responsible sources
FSC® C105338

If you have any concerns about our products,
you can contact us on
ProductSafety@springernature.com

In case Publisher is established outside the EU,
the EU authorized representative is:
Springer Nature Customer Service Center GmbH
Europaplatz 3, 69115 Heidelberg, Germany

Printed by Libri Plureos GmbH
in Hamburg, Germany